Praise for Yoga for Teens

"Yoga 11 has been a class like no other. It has opened my eyes to the practice of yoga and shown me how I can grow physically, mentally, and spiritually.

Throughout the semester, I faced personal challenges, including being honest with myself about certain harmful habits. Through yoga, especially the yamas, I've worked to overcome these obstacles. While I haven't fully climbed all my personal "mountains," I feel hopeful about my future because of what yoga has taught me.

Aside from learning the yamas and niyamas, my favorite part of the class was resting in savasana with a guided mindfulness practice, as it provided deep relaxation for my tired body and my busy mind." ~ A Yoga 11 Student

"I am marking exams — this was my last one. This student has faced significant mental health challenges but has been clean for two years. Yoga has become her anchor. It has truly been life changing. Feeling teary!" ~ A Teacher of Yoga for Teens

"Watching this class grow from a yoga class into a yoga family has been really special. Everyone became so comfortable with each other that we even started saying hi outside of school. Thank you for being such a support this year — I needed it, even in the moments I didn't realize I did." ~ A Student on Favourite Aspects of Yoga 11

"I started high school hoping to have the time of my life. But things quickly went downhill — I became defensive and aggressive, often finding myself in fist fights and weekly confrontations. Life outside of school was also difficult, and I was eventually diagnosed with depression and severe anxiety. I was struggling.

Someone suggested I try yoga, and at first, I thought it was complete nonsense. But I figured adding class, even without free periods, might help keep me out of trouble. In the beginning, I felt foolish and frustrated, and even started skipping classes — but I stuck with it. Over time, I learned how to release the negative energy in my life, to recognize my dreams, and to start working toward them.

Since high school, my life has changed. I've surrounded myself with amazing people, landed a full-time job, and will be starting college next fall.

I can't thank you enough for the impact you've had on my life. Getting up in the morning is no longer a struggle. I'm no longer disappointed to wake up each day — instead, I wake up ready to live." ~ Yoga 11 Student

"This course has and will change many lives, having lasting effects within the education system." ~ Sue Stevenson, Phys. Ed Consultant, NS

"Yoga in Schools fosters the richest learning environment while nurturing character development and total wellness." ~ Jonathan MacKenzie, Yoga 11 Teacher

"You probably get messages like this often, but I wanted to sincerely thank you. I took your yoga class by accident — a scheduling mistake by student services — but looking back, I don't believe it was an accident at all.

Before stepping into your class, I was drowning in self-pity and hatred, blaming those who had hurt me and stolen my happiness. I had made plans to end my life after school, believing I had every reason to do so. But then you shared The Four Agreements with us. One in particular — Don't take things personally — struck something deep within me. At that moment, I realized I had been wasting my life, not truly living it. I was clinging to hurtful words like holding a burning coal, intending to throw it, but only burning myself.

Thank you for giving me the chance to see life through new eyes. I would trade all my years of school just for what I learned in your class: how to feel empathy, offer forgiveness, and find inner peace. With all my gratitude." ~ Yoga 11 Student

"Yoga is more than just exercise — it's a lifestyle. It's breath, flexibility, and strength. It's that feeling you get when you stretch and know your body is thanking you for it. And of course, yoga is fun, too."~ Yoga 11 Student

"Yoga is the place where I can let everything roll off my shoulders and simply not worry. It's a feeling of contentment with myself, a space free of judgment and stereotypes. In yoga, I can truly focus on myself and no one else, because finding my own inner strength is what truly matters." ~ Hannah, YTT Graduate

"I remember the first day I did yoga — something about it immediately caught my interest. I was never someone who enjoyed or excelled in sports, so I feel very fortunate to have found something that offers similar, and even greater, physical benefits while being something I truly enjoy. Yoga has helped me build physical and mental strength, taught me how to live a healthier life, and, most importantly, how to love life." ~ Yoga 11 Student

"Yoga has been one of the best things I've ever done, and I hope to continue with it for years to come. Everything we learned this year has truly helped me." ~ Yoga 11 Student

"At the end of yoga class today I was getting ready for Savasana when a student asked if she could pick a song. I agreed and "Hallelujah" was chosen. The students all laid down and closed their eyes and when KD Lang started singing, so did the entire class of girls. I immediately got goosebumps.

I thought to myself, Savasana is supposed to be a quiet time to look inside oneself and let go, but these students were letting go in their own way. The sound was so beautiful, and the moment was so incredible it brought tears to my eyes.

The only thing I kept thinking was how lucky I was to be teaching this class and that I was the most fortunate teacher in the world. They sang right to the end of the song and at the end, still lying down they clapped in unison for each other.

I was so proud to be teaching such an amazing group of students. When they all sat up, I told them, teary-eyed, that it was the most beautiful Savasana I had ever experienced and expressed how lucky I was to be their teacher. Then we all stood up and gave each other a big group hug. And the first people I wanted to share this with were you, my teachers, Jenny and Blair. Namaste." ~ Letter from a Yoga 11 High School Teacher

Yoga for Teens

A Mindful Guide for Helping Teens Cultivate Calm, Strength, and Resilience

JENNY KEIRSTEAD

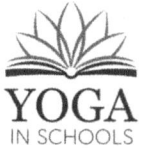

YOGA
IN SCHOOLS

Copyright © 2025 by Jenny Maria Kierstead

Published by Breathing Space Yoga under the imprint Yoga Books

All Rights Reserved. Except for use in any review, no part of this book may be reproduced, stored in a retrieval system, or transmit-ted in any form or by any means, electronic, mechanical, or otherwise, without written permission from the publisher.

Cover and Interior Design by Woven Red Author Services, www.WovenRed.ca
Cover and stock images used with permission via www.depositphotos.com

Asana images © Jenny Kierstead

Yoga for Teens/Jenny Kierstead—1st edition
ISBN paperback: 978-0-9953409-8-5
ISBN electronic PDF: 978-0-9953409-9-2

Contact Jenny and Blair at:
info@YogainSchools.ca
www.YogaInSchools.ca
1 (902)-444-9642

Dedication

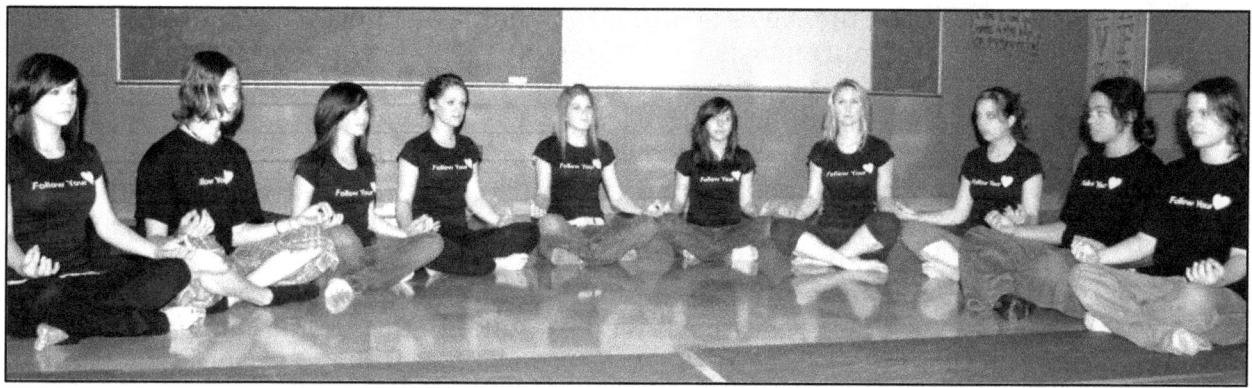

This manual is dedicated to all adolescents, struggling to embrace their true self. This photo is of the first Yoga 11 class in 2005.

This revised and updated edition is dedicated to Lisa McCully — educator, mother, and sister of *Yoga in Schools* founder, Jenny Kierstead. Lisa's life was tragically taken in the 2020 mass casualty, shortly after completing her master's degree in education, where she focused on virtues-based leadership.

It was Lisa who first introduced Jenny to yoga in their twenties, while they were living together in Vancouver, BC. Years later, during her own Yoga Teacher Training with Jenny and Blair, Lisa contributed to the development of this manual by assisting with the assessment segment. Her passion for children, education, and higher learning continues to echo through these teachings, gently guiding us all toward a more peaceful and compassionate world.

Finally, it is with deep gratitude to the pioneers and practitioners of Yoga that we share this manual. May this body of work honor their dedication and hard-earned wisdom. We acknowledge Jenny's late teacher, **Shri K. Pattabhi Jois**, who was instrumental in bringing the Ashtanga Yoga system from Mysore, India, to the wider world. We also recognize the dedication of his daughter **Saraswati** and his grandson, **Sharath Jois**, whose stewardship and lifelong devotion to the yoga tradition inspired students across generations.

A Message from the Author

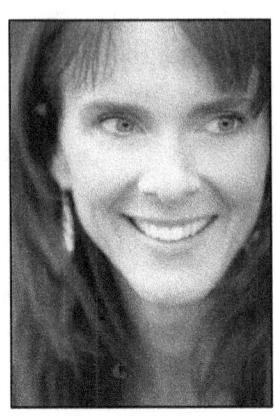

After receiving numerous emails from our yoga teacher graduates seeking more detailed guidance on the Yoga 11 curriculum I created for the Nova Scotia Department of Education, it became clear that a comprehensive set of lesson plans was needed to better support the dedicated educators bringing yoga and mindfulness into classrooms.

Compiling these lessons has allowed me to expand on the exercises and activities we cover in our yoga teacher training program, offering greater clarity and structure. This manual is designed to help you share the rich, timeless teachings of yoga with today's youth in a way that is both meaningful and accessible.

In this latest edition, I've incorporated content from several of our other programs as well—including the *Mindfulness in Schools Manual*, *Trauma-Sensitive Mindfulness*, *Anxiety Recovery*, *Girl on Fire Empowerment*, *Yoga for Autism*, and *Yoga for Diverse Learners*. My hope is that this added variety will deepen your impact and further support your students' growth, resilience, and well-being.

We are living through an extraordinary time of transformation. I believe passionately in contributing to this global shift in consciousness by empowering the next generation—our teens—to lead the way forward. For this transformation to take root, we must guide them with intention and care.

Let's show them a new way of being—one that invites a profound shift:
- From victimhood to accountability
- From material preoccupations to meaningful connection
- From harmful habits to holistic self-care
- From a culture of hate to one of kindness and compassion

By creating space for students to reflect on how they treat themselves and others, we can help them cultivate inner peace, vibrant health, and the life skills they need to positively shape the world around them.

Thank you for your commitment to educating the next generation. It is truly one of the most important investments we can make. I also hope that in the midst of supporting others, you take time to reflect on your own journey and care for yourself with the same compassion you offer your students.

With gratitude,

Jenny

Other Work by Jenny Kierstead

Yoga Posters: Yoga 1 (Elementary) and Yoga 2 (Secondary) Posters, with accompanying manuals and cross-curricular suggestions

Breathing Space Yoga Teacher Training Manual, (250 pages)

Mindfulness in Schools Manual, (220 pages) co-written with Blair Abbass

Yoga for Autism, co-written with Catherine Rahey

Yoga for Diverse Learners

Girl on Fire Empowerment Manual

Girl on Fire Mother-Daughter Journal

Trauma-Sensitive Mindfulness and Yoga Training

Anxiety Recovery Training and Personal Journey

Qigong Teacher Training

Gratitude

Thank you to the many teachers who have been putting these lessons to the test and for passing along students' growth experiences over the years.

I give thanks to our youth for opening their minds and hearts to receive these teachings, and for being willing to carry them forward.

Many thanks to the amazing teens who demonstrated the 50 foundational asanas within this manual:

- Daniella Attedjro
- Omar Eberham
- Bella Kierstead-Abbass
- Sophia Kierstead-Abbass
- Princess Samou
- Sydney Steeves
- Oliva Wilkinson
- Regan Woodsworth

We recognize the professional editors, Nibedita Sen and Kevin Pearle, who put final touches on this manual.

We also have deep gratitude for Joan Frantschuk, who spent countless hours bringing this manual to completion through her fine formatting and organizational skills.

A special thanks to our daughter Bella (16 at the time), who directed the photo shoot, in her organized and humorous fashion.

Finally, my deepest gratitude goes to my husband and business partner, Blair, for seeing the vision of Yoga in Schools and for creating so many opportunities for me to share my passions.

Jenny

Land Acknowledgement (from Nova Scotia)

Let's begin with a few grounding breaths.

Feel your body supported by the floor beneath you, and the floor held by this beautiful, intelligent Earth.

I invite us all to take a moment to honour the ancestral lands on which we reside.

We acknowledge that we are in Mi'kma'ki (MEEG-MA-GEE), the traditional and unceded territory of the Mi'kmaq people.

We also recognize and honour the enduring presence of people of African descent in Nova Scotia, whose history on this land spans over 400 years.

Let us honour the ancient roots of yoga and the wisdom tradition from which it comes—the land and people of India.

May our time on the mat today nurture a world grounded in kindness, equity, respect, and safety for all.

Shanti, Shanti, Shanti — Peace, Peace, Peace.

Namaste — the light in me honours the light in you.

(*Feel free to close with any culturally meaningful or respectful greeting of your choice.*)

Table of Contents

How To Use These Lessons ... 1

Weekly Planner ... 2

Long Term Goals ... 4

Daily Participation Evaluation ... 5
   Participation Rubric ... 5
   Participation Assessment ... 6

Daily Lesson Plan #1: Welcome to Yoga 11 ... 9
   Note to Parents of Yoga 11 Students ... 10
   Yoga Title Page ... 11
      Yoga Title Page Rubric ... 11
   Yoga Class Agreement ... 11
      1. Be Respectful ... 11
      2. Be Present ... 11
      3. Be Safe ... 11
      4. Be Intentional ... 12
      5. Group-Generated Agreements ... 12

Daily Lesson Plan #2: Introduction to Yoga ... 13
   History of Yoga and Sanskrit ... 14
   Charging Your Inner Batteries ... 15
   Handout: Wellness Portfolio Explained ... 16

Daily Lesson Plan #3: Life of a Yogi ... 17
   Life of a Yogi ... 18
      A Snapshot of a Yogi in Optimal Health ... 18
   Is Yoga a Religion? ... 19

Daily Lesson Plan #4: Natural Breath ... 20
   Breathing Log ... 21

Daily Lesson Plan #5: Breathing Flow ... 22
   Namaste Definition ... 23
      Curriculum Outcomes ... 23

Daily Lesson Plan #6: Namaste ... 24
   Koshas – The Layers of the Self ... 25
      Annamaya Kosha ... 25
      Pranamaya Kosha ... 25
      Manomaya and Vijnanamaya Koshas ... 26
      Anandamaya Kosha ... 26

Daily Lesson Plan #7: Mountain Introduction 27
Mountain – Tadasana / Samasthiti Benefits of Practicing Proper Posture 28
Mountain – Tadasana / Samasthiti 28
Optional Pre-Activity 28
Mountain / Tadasana – Peer Evaluation 30
Teaching Points Checklist for Tadasana 30

Daily Lesson Plan #8: Mountain in Motion 31
Posture Alignment Rubric 32
Curriculum Outcomes 33
Posture Observation Chart 33
Mountain Reflection 33
Journal Prompts 33
Closing Reflection 33

Daily Lesson Plan #9: Mountain Mindfulness Practice 34
Script for Teacher to Read 34
Ask yourself 35
Follow-Up Suggestions 35
Student Reflection Questions 35

Daily Lesson Plan #10: Sun Salutation A/Surya Namaskar A 36
Surya Namaskar: The Complete Practice 37
Energy of Sun Salutations 38
Sun Breath & Sun Salutation A/Surya Namaskar A Scripts 38
Ancient Wisdom, Modern Relevance 38
Sun Breath Script: 38
Modified Sun Salutation/Surya Namaskar A Script: 39
Complete Sun Salutation/Surya Namaskar A Script 39

Daily Lesson Plan #11: Sun Salutation B/Surya Namaskar B 40
Surya Namaskar B – Sun Salutation B Script 41
Affirmation 41
Sequence 41
Benefits of Sun Salutation B 42
Physical 42
Energetic 43

Daily Lesson Plan #12: Breathing Styles 44
The Effects of Yoga on the Nervous System 44
Yoga: More Than Physical Fitness 44
Understanding the Nervous System 45
The Stress Response: Fight, Flight, or Freeze 45
The Relaxation Response: Rest and Digest 45
Why This Matters 46
Teaching Tip 46
The Four Types of Yoga 46
1. Jnana Yoga – The Yoga of Wisdom 46
2. Bhakti Yoga – The Yoga of Devotion 46

    3. Karma Yoga – The Yoga of Action 47
    4. Raja Yoga – The Yoga of the Mind 47
    Reflection 48
  Namaskar Project 48
    Curriculum Outcomes 48
    Project Instructions 48
    Steps to Complete 48
    Alignment Rubric 49

Daily Lesson Plan #13: Four Types of Yoga 50
  Affirmations on Yamas 51
  Karma Yoga – The Path of Selfless Service 51
    A Real-Life Reflection 51
    Examples in the Community 52
    What Karma Yoga Teaches Us 52
    Living the Karma Yoga Way 52
    A Personal Invitation 52

Daily Lesson Plan #14: Yamas and Niyamas 53
  Giving New Light to a Dark Day 54
    A Mission of Love 54
    A Ripple of Positivity 55
    Your Turn: Practicing Ahimsa 55
    What's Your Plan? 55

Daily Lesson Plan #15: Peace Project 56
  Proposal and Planning Process 57
    Brainstorm 57
    Get Approval 57
    Design a Form to Display the Following Information 57
    Sketch a Rough Draft of Your Form 58
    Your Reflection 58
  Reflection Guidelines: Sharing Your Experience 59
    1. Purpose and Vision 59
    2. Collaboration and Teamwork (if applicable) 59
    3. Personal Highlights and Emotions 59
    4. Challenges and Lessons Learned 59
    5. Gratitude and Acknowledgments 59
    6. Community Impact 59
    Final Note 60
    Sample Reflection on Project Hug: Compassion into Action 60
  Peace Project Rubric 61
  Peace Project Assessment 61

Daily Lesson Plan #16: Knowing & Speaking Your Truth/Satya 63
  Classical Namaskar/Salutation Script 64
    Right Side 64
    Left Side 65
  Article: Moment of Truth 65

    Illusion and Awakening..65

Daily Lesson Plan #17: Non-Stealing/Honesty/Asteya 67
    Article on Asteya-Non-Stealing/Honesty 68
        Asteya Affirmation & Reflection Activity 68
        Asteya Affirmation 69
        Let's Reflect 69
        The Second Half of the Affirmation 69
        From Guilt to Generosity 69

Daily Lesson Plan #18: Energy Management/Brahmacharya 70
    Understanding Brahmacharya: Energy, Moderation, and Respect 71

Daily Lesson Plan #19: Generosity/Aparigraha 73
    Aparigraha: The Art of Letting Go 74
    Beyond Minimalism 74
    How Aparigraha Shows Up in Daily Life 74
    Practicing Aparigraha 75
    Living With Open Hands 75

Daily Lesson Plan #20: Review of Yamas 76
        Yama Creative Assignment 77
        Reflection Journal Entry (Written Component) 77
        Creative Component (Art Piece) 77
    Yama Rubric 78

Daily Lesson Plan #21: Introduction to Niyamas and Purity/Saucha 79
    Transforming Toxic Relationships with Saucha, Q & A with Jenny and Blair 80
        Question 80
        Blair 80
        Jenny 81

Daily Lesson Plan #22: Contentment/Santosha 82
    The Grip 83

Daily Lesson Plan #23: Balancing Effort/Sthira and Ease/Sukha 84

Daily Lesson Plan #24: Igniting Heat/Tapas 86
    Igniting Your Inner Flame: Cultivating Tapas 87
    Practice and Tapas (Self-Discipline) 88

Daily Lesson Plan #25: Self-reflection/Swadhyaya 89
    The Importance of Self-Reflection 90

Daily Lesson Plan #26: Self-Study/Swadhyaya and Sacred Texts 92

Daily Lesson Plan #27: Belief in love/Ishvara Pranidhana 93

Daily Lesson Plan #28: Review of Niyamas 95
The First Two Limbs in Review (20 points) 96
Yamas 96
Niyamas 96

Daily Lesson Plan #29: The Mindful Limbs of Raja Yoga 98
Dopamine versus Oxytocin 99
Mindfulness Journal Reflection 100

Daily Lesson Plan #30: The Eight Limbs Creative Art Piece 101

Daily Lesson Plan #31: Letting Go Ritual 103
Sample Letter to Your Current Self 104

Daily Lesson Plan #32: Intention Setting 1 105
Today, I'll see my life as if it's brand new 107

Daily Lesson Plan #33: Intention Setting 2 108
The Wheel of Life 109

Daily Lesson Plan #34: Food as Medicine 110
Mindfulness Raisin Practice 110
The Yoga of Eating 111
Brainstorm 111
What do you think that means? 112
Which foods wouldn't fit into this category? 112
Reflect 112

Daily Lesson Plan #35: Ritual of Food 113

Daily Lesson Plan #36: Anatomy of Asanas 115
Anatomy: The Skeletal and Muscular Systems 116
The Skeletal System 116
Bone Shapes 116
Anatomy of an Asana Assignment 118
Curriculum Outcomes 118
Assignment Overview 118
Steps to Complete the Assignment 118
Citation Guidelines 119
Anatomy of an Asana Rubric 119
Anatomy of an Asana Assessment 120

Daily Lesson Plan #37: Researching Systems 122
Systems of the Body 122
The Systems of the Body 122
Peer-Assessment for Systems Presentation 123

Daily Lesson Plan #38: Presentations 124

    The Ego versus the Self 124

Daily Lesson Plan #39: Internal/SELF-Referenced Living 126
    The Treasure Within 127
    Questions to go with Treasure Story 127

Daily Lesson Plan #40: Yoga Flow Design 129
    Yoga Class Outline Handout: 20-minute Peer-Led Practice Teaching Class 130
    Practice Teaching Guideline 132
        Curriculum Outcomes 132
        Assignment Overview 132
        Playlist Requirements 132
        Suggested Class Structure 132

Daily Lesson Plan #41: Yoga Class Presentations 133
    Peer Assessment Handout 134
    Chakra Handout 135

Daily Lesson Plan #42: Student Teaching 136
    Asana Flow Chart 136
        Asana Sequence Assignment Instructions 136
        Asana Chart 138
    Practice Teaching Reflection 139

Daily Lesson Plan #43: Yoga Class in Nature 140
    Reconnecting with Nature 141

Daily Lesson Plan #44: Yin Yoga for Self-love 142

Daily Lesson Plan #45: Girl on Fire Empowerment Class 145

Daily Lesson Plan #46: Yoga for Autism Energizing Class 146

Daily Lesson Plan #47: Yoga for Diverse Learners, Happy Feet Class 149

Daily Lesson Plan #48: Trauma-sensitive Movement Practice 151

Daily Lesson Plan #49 Anxiety Calming Movement Practice 153

Daily Lesson Plan #50: Wrap up 154
    Game of Jeopardy 154
    Yoga 11 Worksheet 155
        Origins and Philosophy 155
        Physical Practice 155
        Mindfulness 156
        Personal Reflection 156
    Breathing Practices included in this Manual 157
        Teaching Considerations 157

    Breathing Practices Overview 158
50 Foundational Asanas 159
    Mindfulness Asanas 160
    Standing Asanas 160
    Standing Balance Asanas 161
    Arm Balance Asanas 161
    Inversions 162
    Backbending Asanas 162
    Seated Asanas 162
    Core Strengthening Asanas 163
    Hip Opening Asanas 163
    Twisting Asanas 164
    Closing Asanas 164

Yoga for Teens

How To Use These Lessons

Each lesson plan is organized in a sequence that gradually introduces asanas (postures) and key concepts, increasing in depth and intensity as the course progresses. However, you are encouraged to adapt the sequence to best suit the unique needs of your student population.

Many lessons contain enough material to span two class sessions, so this should be taken into account when planning your term. It's recommended that you read through the entire manual before beginning, to get a clear sense of what can realistically be covered based on your time allocation, class size, and teaching context.

Weekly Planner

This weekly planner is intended to help structure lessons or activities on a weekly basis across a typical month.

Things to include might be:
- Lesson plans to cover each day
- Important dates or goals
- Assignments

For the Week of:
Monday:
Tuesday:
Wednesday:
Thursday:
Friday:
Method of Evaluation:

Weekly Planner

Outcomes:

Outcomes:

Long Term Goals

Supplementary Materials required:

Outcomes for this Section:

Guest Speakers:

Methods of Evaluation:

Subject:
Class:
Term 1:
Term 2:

Daily Participation Evaluation

Participation Rubric

FREQUENCY	POINTS
RARELY	0-1
SOMETIMES	2
OFTEN	3
ALMOST ALWAYS	4
ALWAYS	5

ATTRIBUTE	REQUIREMENT
PUNCTUALITY	Student arrives to class on time.
PREPARED FOR LEARNING	Student arrives to class wearing appropriate clothing, with binder and journal.
PARTICIPATION	Student is fully engaged and requires no prompting to participate.
RESPECT FOR CLASSROOM	Student shows respect for classmates, space, and equipment.
DISCIPLINED EFFORT	Student strives for proper alignment and breathing in asanas, working within their growing edge.
YOGA ETIQUETTE	Student practices Yamas (ethical disciplines) & Niyamas (personal observances).
MINDFULNESS	Student practices screen-free self-awareness and presence throughout the class

Participation Assessment

STUDENT NAME:	PUNCTUALITY	PREPARED FOR LEARNING	PARTICIPATION	RESPECT FOR CLASSROOM	DISCIPLINED EFFORT	YOGA ETIQUETTE	MINDFULNESS	TOTAL
DATE:				CLASS:				
1								
2								
3								
4								
5								
6								
7								
8								
9								
10								
11								
12								
13								

Daily Participation Evaluation

14									
15									
16									
17									
18									
19									
20									
21									
22									
23									
24									

Daily Lesson Plan #1: Welcome to Yoga 11

Intention/Objective
Introduce students to the practice and philosophy of Yoga through the opening Yoga sutra 1.1 "And now, the practice of Yoga begins." This new beginning can be discussed and posted on the wall or written on the board. Students will apply the Yoga Class Agreement to their own practice.
Review/Introduction
Nametags: Students can draw or print a symbol that reflects who they are as individuals. Share your symbol with a friend or neighbor in twos or threes.
Lesson
Housekeeping: <ul><li>Outline daily routine (Find a mat, blocks, band and eye pillow, find a spot, finish class by wiping down mat etc).</li><li>Class Outline will be on this wall each day.</li><li>Washroom locations.</li><li>Importance of participation.</li><li>Readiness (you may realize you're not).</li><li>Phone basket, where phones live during the entire class.</li><li>Discuss the unique nature of the course-that it will be unlike any other they've attended in school. Although there will be discussion time and personal reflective opportunities, this is in no way a bird course. In fact, many find this more challenging than other courses because it calls us to be fully present in an honest and compassionate way.</li><li>Discuss the letter to parents.</li><li>Discuss the Yoga Class Agreement.</li><li>Explain trauma-sensitive terms that will be used: instead of 'positions' or 'poses' we'll be referring to body postures, forms, shapes or asanas.</li></ul>
Reflection/Conclusion
Savasana while exploring with the idea of deepening your breath and softening tension.
OMwork
<ul><li>Give the letter to your parents to sign and return.</li><li>Design a title page that symbolizes the beginning of your yogic journey, which can include symbols, words, aspirations and intentions.</li></ul>
OMwork Material
<ul><li>Note to Parents</li><li>Yoga Title Page Rubric</li><li>Daily Participation Rubric</li><li>Yoga Class Agreement</li></ul>

Daily Lesson Plan #1:
Welcome to Yoga 11

Note to Parents of Yoga 11 Students

Date:

Dear Parent(s)/Guardian(s),

I'm reaching out to let you know that your child has enrolled in the *PE Yoga 11* course this term. The purpose of this letter is to provide you with an overview of the course, including material requirements and the nature of the yoga practice.

Below is an excerpt from the course curriculum:

> *Yoga 11* introduces students to the practice of yoga. With its profound ability to support vibrant physical, mental, and emotional health, the goal is for students to cultivate a lifelong yoga practice. This supports not only physical well-being but also nurtures positive relationships with themselves, others, and the natural world.

Students will engage in a variety of activities, including physical postures (asanas), personal reflection, partner exercises, and classroom-based theory. The physical component of yoga emphasizes strength, flexibility, balance, and breath control—all of which contribute to overall health and enhance performance in other physical activities. The mental component supports focus, emotional regulation, and stress reduction by calming the nervous system.

Classroom sessions will explore a range of topics such as the fundamentals of good nutrition, core ethical principles (including kindness, generosity, and respect), and practices that empower students to become thoughtful, engaged members of society.

Minimal equipment is needed. All yoga props will be provided. However, for sanitary reasons, your child may wish to bring their own yoga mat. A journal or notebook is required, along with a binder for organizing assignments into a wellness portfolio, which will be submitted at the end of the course.

Students are encouraged to wear comfortable, flexible clothing that allows for a full range of movement. A more fitted style is often preferred to ensure coverage during various postures.

If you have any questions or concerns throughout the term, please feel free to reach out via phone or email.

Warmly,

Parent's Signature: _____

Parent's Name: _____

Parent's email: _____

Yoga Title Page

Curriculum Outcomes

Design a title page that symbolizes the beginning of your yogic journey, which can include symbols, words, aspirations, and intentions.
- Students will be expected to apply their understanding of yogic text and principles to their daily lives & yoga practice.
- Students will be expected to apply the principles of yoga in a personal way outside of yoga practice.

Yoga Title Page Rubric

ACHIEVEMENT	POINTS
Student met partial requirements	1
Students met requirements with satisfaction	2
Students met requirements with excellence	3

Yoga Class Agreement

This agreement supports the creation of a respectful, supportive, and mindful space for all participants. These guiding principles can be reviewed at the start of each session to help establish a positive group culture.

1. Be Respectful

- Honor each participant's personal mat space.
- Maintain confidentiality: whatever is shared in the yoga classroom stays within the group.

2. Be Present

- Arrive on time, prepared to engage fully.
- Place phones in the designated basket to minimize distractions.
- Commit to being mentally and emotionally present throughout practice.

3. Be Safe

- Practice interoception: listen to your body's signals and respect your personal "Growing Edge" (where 1 = fully disengaged, and 10 = overwhelmed with intensity). Aim to practice within a range of 4–7.
- Contribute to a safe space for others through non-judgment, acceptance, and tolerance.

4. Be Intentional

- At the beginning of each practice, set a personal intention that reflects your current needs and goals.

5. Group-Generated Agreements

- Collaboratively brainstorm and add additional agreements that students feel will support a positive and meaningful yoga experience.

"Yoga is 99% practice and 1% theory." - Sri K. Pattabhi Jois

Daily Lesson Plan #2: Introduction to Yoga

Intention/Objective
Introduction to Yoga.
Teaching Resource Material
History of Yoga and Sanskrit Handout
Review/Introduction
<ul><li>Submit title page and signed letter from parents.</li><li>Natural Breathing for 5 min with soothing music.</li><li>Lie on your back, close your eyes and notice your breathing. Allow the breath to soften areas of tension or stress. Feel your body melt into your mat like warm butter on toast. With each breath, continue softening, and letting go.</li><li>Proceed through guided relaxation with auto suggestion (naming various body parts to relax).</li></ul>
Lesson
Brief Movement Practice<ul><li>Start on your back, with Knee to Chest/Apanasana by bringing your right knee to your chest with your left leg resting on the mat, open your right leg out right, crossover into a supine twist, back to center and straighten the right leg to the ceiling with fingers interlocked around your thigh or calf.</li><li>Circle foot in one direction, then to the other, then point and flex. Lift head to knee and walk the hands up toward the heel, feel the core engage.</li><li>Inhale and lower the head, exhale, release the leg slowly down and take a few breaths to observe sensations before switching sides.</li><li>Half Bridge position, as the hips lift, the arms stretch overhead alongside the ears and exhale, then lower the hips, along with the arms.</li><li>Roll to one side, rise slowly to sitting and take a moment to notice how you feel after just a few stretches.</li></ul>**Brainstorm**<ul><li>"What is Yoga?" Have students share the first thing that comes to mind, record their answers on chart paper so they can be added to later in the unit.</li><li>Yoga means Yuj, to yoke, unite or bind. Why do you think the body, mind, spirit connection is so important? This is the uniting essence behind Yoga. Read yoga sutra 1.2.</li><li>Refer to handout on the history of yoga for a brief definition and to the Breathing Space Yoga Manual for an expanded definition.</li><li>Discuss Sanskrit terms with open discussion on English equivalents.</li><li>Introduce the Bandha System, letting them discover their transverse abdominis/Uddiyana Bandha by pressing index and middle fingers inside of hip bones and moving the belly away from fingers.</li></ul>
Reflection/Conclusion
Review the Sanskrit terms and ask them to walk out with their Bandhas engaged.

Daily Lesson Plan #2:
Introduction to Yoga

OMwork
• Imagine how the concept of yoga, coming together in peace, could transform the world as we know it. What might be different on a personal level and global level? • Research the term Prana, which is used frequently in the yoga classroom and record definitions. Fill out the handout on Prana and submit it the next day. • Start building your wellness portfolio by adding your Omwork to it.
OMwork Material
• Charging your inner batteries • Wellness Portfolio Description

History of Yoga and Sanskrit

Yoga began 5,000 years ago in India as a practice for young men in training to be sages or wise men. The postures, known as asanas, strengthened their bodies so that they could sit for lengthy periods of time in mindfulness practice to expand their understanding of life. The asanas also helped to harmonize the systems of their bodies. A strong body enabled their minds to rest in the present moment and their consciousness to rise above the fear-based limits of our conditioned perspective, into a state of unity, love and peace.

When it began, yoga was practiced by men in the pursuit of personal mastery, while the women raised the family. Now, with the current work and family demands on all genders today, yoga has become a tool to mitigate the damaging effects of stress, cultivate peace and transform the body into a healthy, flexible and strong machine. Today, our goals are a bit more practical than our 'forefathers', with many practitioners reporting they do yoga to build core strength or repair their standing posture or learn tools to de-stress or recover their natural breathing rhythm.

The ancient language of yoga is Sanskrit, one of the first known languages ever created alongside other intricate indigenous languages. Each asana and gesture have a Sanskrit name that will become a part of your practice throughout the course. You're encouraged to notice how you feel when you hear or speak the language of Sanskrit, as it was developed by people who'd devoted their lives to connecting to the powerful healing energies of the natural world.

The most used Sanskrit terms: Yoga, Asana, Vinyasa, Bandha, OM, Shanti, Namaste

Yoga: Translates from Sanskrit into yoke or union. One of the most used descriptions of yoga is the uniting of body/mind/spirit. Yoga is a process of learning what it means to discover true happiness, health and contentment by living a life of virtue and goodness. The practice of yoga empowers us to examine our lifestyle choices and to make decisions that support our wellbeing, and respect others.

Asana: A Sanskrit term referring to a body shape that is held for a period (typically 5-7 breaths), with both strength and ease.

Vinyasa translates to "to place in a special way", reflected in the mindful movement of asanas coordinated with the breath, which are linked together in yoga practice. Vinyasa also refers to the short connecting sequences used in Ashtanga and Flow classes, moving from Chaturanga Dandasana (Low Staff Pose) to Urdhva Mukha Svanasana (Upward Dog Pose) to Adho Mukha Svanasana (Downward Dog Pose). This short sequence is done between asanas to maintain heat and stamina.

Bandha: Intentional muscular contractions, used to cultivate energy in our core and restore balance in our vital organs. It can be seen as a valve, which harnesses life force energy, without restraining the necessary flow of certain energies.

OM: The OM (English) or AUM (Sanskrit) is a symbol of unity, or oneness. It is known to be similar to the most basic primordial sounds of the universe and is said to be one of the most healing sound frequencies.

Shanti: A mantra is a vocal sound spoken with a focused intent, with the understanding that our thoughts and intentions shape our reality. OM Shanti Shanti Shanti, a mantra that invokes peace, is often chanted to close a class. It is used as a reminder that the peace cultivated in our practice is always accessible and that our role as yogis is to be ambassadors for peace.

Shanti is usually chanted with hands together, your first shanti can be chanted with thumbs at the brow, to symbolize peace in our minds, the second shanti can be spoken with thumbs at the lips, encouraging us to spread peace with our words and the third shanti can be done with hands at heart centre, reminding us to live with peace in our hearts. You could also explain before the chanting of the three Shanti's that the first one will be chanted for us, the next one for our loved ones and the last one for the entire world.

Namaste: There are many translations of this powerful greeting. As a class you will come up with a translation that everyone agrees upon to close each class (including hands at heart- Anjali mudra). A simple translation is "The light in me recognizes and honors the light in you."

Charging Your Inner Batteries

Lifestyle choices that deplete Prana/energy (what drains your body battery)	Lifestyle choices that fuel Prana/energy (what charges your body battery)

Daily Lesson Plan #2:
Introduction to Yoga

Handout: Wellness Portfolio Explained

As part of the Yoga 11 assessment structure, you will be compiling your reflections, Omwork pieces and teaching assignments into a portfolio, which will contribute to your final mark. You can choose to compile hard copies of your assignments OR create a digital portfolio. Other than the teacher having access to these assignments for marking your participation, nobody else will be reading these items. The hope is that when you have completed the course, you will have a compilation of skills, memories, and insights for you to keep.

Daily Lesson Plan #3: Life of a Yogi

Intention/Objective
Introduce students to the attitude and practices of a yogic lifestyle.
Review/Introduction
<ul><li>Discuss their reflections on the term yoga and the things that drain their batteries and charge their batteries.</li><li>Today we will gain even more clarity on what a yogic lifestyle entails.</li></ul>
Lesson
Centering:<ul><li>Lie down and revisit yogic breathing, slowing the pace and filling the lungs entirely, followed by a complete exhalation.</li><li>Review the Yoga Class Agreement</li><li>Take a moment to create an intention for your class, a reason for being here or perhaps hold a question in mind that you'd like the answer to.</li></ul>**Body of Class:**<ul><li>Reach arms overhead, stretching through the right side, then left, making the body as long as possible.</li><li>Tuck both knees into chest and rock from side to side, relax the head on the mat.</li><li>Right knee stays tucked into the chest, while the left extends along the floor.</li><li>Proceed into Half Anada Balasanda with the right hand at the arch.</li><li>Straighten the right leg, pressing the heel to the sky with fingers interlocked behind the thigh. Lift nose to knee then let the arms go, reaching toward the left foot to awaken the core. Hold your leg upright for 3 breaths and lower down slowly. Do the same on the left side.</li><li>Rise to sitting and undulate the spine (arch/round) in the Jellyfish, finding your Bandha/abdominal engagement on the exhalation. Fun fact: Jellyfish have no bones or blood, but they do have a nervous system. Can you nurture your NS now with a slow, deep breath?</li><li>Cross the feet and come into Hero/Virasana, 5 breaths.</li><li>Table, continue with the arching and rounding movement of the spine.</li><li>Explore Balancing Table, add bind if possible.</li><li>Modified side plank with lower knee on the mat or top foot grounded. Circle the top arm 2 times and reach it overhead, stretching the side waist. Other side.</li><li>Back to Table, walk hands slightly forward and lower down into chaturanga dandasana.</li><li>Cobra with hands lifted (feet anchored) to activate spinal muscles, 3 times.</li><li>Downward Dog for five breaths.</li><li>Lunge forward with right foot, transition to the left by scissoring the legs a few times in midair and landing in a lunge on the left side.</li><li>Step forward to Seaweed (standing forward fold) and rise slowly, methodically stacking one vertebra over the other, gradually coming to an upright Mountain form.</li><li>Observe the way you feel, standing with 'proper posture'. Does this reflect your usual stance?</li></ul>**Closing:**<ul><li>Take a seat and close your eyes or downcast your gaze while the teacher and/or various students read the Life of a Yogi hand out. What stood out for you as inspiring, strange or brand new?</li></ul>

• Briefly discuss the attitudes and practices of a yogic lifestyle that were developed 5,000 years ago.
Reflection/Conclusion
The Life of a Yogi demonstrates the components of holistic health and self-care that will be explored and studied throughout the course.
OMwork
• Read through the 'The Life of a Yogi' on your own time and create an intention to embrace one or two aspects of this description that you currently do not live but aspire toward. What stood out for you as important? • Record your reflections in your journal and add your intentions into your wellness portfolio.
OMwork Material
• Life of a Yogi Handout • Is Yoga a Religion? Handout

Life of a Yogi

A Snapshot of a Yogi in Optimal Health

Take a moment to reflect: are any of the following part of your daily experience?

Physical:

- You wake up with a smile, feeling refreshed and energized after a peaceful, uninterrupted night of sleep.
- You prioritize quality rest, aiming for 8–10 hours of deep, restorative sleep each night.
- You appreciate and care for the body you've been given, knowing it is your lifelong home.
- You experience regular, effortless bowel movements as a natural part of your day.
- You treat your body with respect, engaging in consistent movement that builds strength, flexibility, and stamina.
- You enjoy a healthy relationship with your body and weight, addressing hormone imbalances or making dietary adjustments as needed to support a vibrant life.
- You nourish your body with wholesome foods: fresh fruits, vegetables, whole grains, eggs, nuts, seeds, fish, and poultry. Most days, you eat when you're hungry and stop when you're full.
- You stay attuned to your body's cues—responding to thirst with clean, pure water.

Mental:

- You laugh often—those deep, belly laughs that leave your face sore and your spirit lifted.
- Your intimate relationships are rooted in mutual respect, care, and consideration.
- You see yourself as equally deserving of love and respect as everyone else—no more, no less.
- You use discernment to invite emotionally healthy and kind individuals into your inner circle.
- You set healthy screen boundaries that align with your goals and passions, choosing entertainment that reflects your values and inspires your best self.

- Your ability to focus comes naturally, thanks to nourishing lifestyle choices that support your brain and nervous system.
- Your daily yoga and mindfulness practice creates a calming, grounded presence that others can trust and rely on.
- You maintain strong and steady mental health, approaching life's challenges with calm, rational thought and deep trust in your resilience.

Spiritual:

- You have a passion for learning and growing, pursuing experiences and knowledge that inspire you. In turn, you joyfully share your unique gifts with the world.
- Your self-confidence empowers you to be authentically yourself, regardless of outside opinions or judgment.
- You focus your energy on personal growth and meaningful contribution, protecting your attention from harmful influences and unnecessary distractions.
- Your self-care habits and rituals sustain your energy without the need for stimulants like caffeine, sugar, or vaping.
- You trust your instincts and intuition, developed through daily time on your mat and quiet reflection—deeply connected to your boundaries.

Write your own ideal life situation that reflects health, happiness, purpose and success.

Is Yoga a Religion?

Yoga is not a religion, though its strong ethical foundations may resemble those found in many religious traditions. Rather, it is a way of life—a holistic approach to living—with the central aim of becoming a better human being through practices such as kindness, honesty, and generosity.

Because these values are shared across many spiritual and religious paths, yoga can serve as a powerful complement to one's existing beliefs and traditions. In addition to its moral and philosophical components, yoga is widely practiced for its physical and mental health benefits, including stress reduction, increased strength and flexibility, and disease prevention—benefits accessible to people of all faiths and backgrounds.

Yoga integrates both theory and physical movement, engaging the mind and body together. It invites us to embark on a personal journey of transformation by deepening our self-awareness and our understanding of our place in the world. As our perspective broadens, we begin to see ourselves not as isolated beings, but as individual expressions of a greater whole—like single waves rising from the same vast ocean of creation.

How might you use your yoga practice to deepen your connection to your existing beliefs and rituals?

Daily Lesson Plan #4: Natural Breath

Intention/Objective
Students will demonstrate an understanding of the natural breath and the most common restorative body form, Savasana. **Note**: If the room is usually quite cool, arrive early to turn the heat up for this class.
Teaching Resource Material
<ul><li>Eye pillows for each student (Perhaps invite elderly people to make these in advance).</li><li>Feathers for each student.</li><li>Note to teacher: the breathing instruction below is a trauma-informed approach, gently guiding the breath deeper and deeper.</li></ul>
Review/Introduction
Present your Title Page to a partner or to a small group, explaining the content. Discuss in partners the aspect of the life of a yogi that you've chosen to focus on.
Lesson
Centering:<ul><li>Re-discovering the Natural Breath:</li><li>The term 'Re-discovering' is used because at the beginning of our lives, we all breathed naturally, and deeply. As life happens, with its heartbreak, criticisms and self-doubt, we instinctively hold or shorten the breath to protect ourselves from pain. This causes many health concerns, such as anxiety, stress, digestive dysfunctions, cardiovascular issues etc.</li><li>Brainstorm ways in which the breath is altered to deal with life's challenges (withholding, huffing and puffing, shallow breathing etc).</li></ul>**Body of class:**<ul><li>Seated Easy Asana/Sukhasana with the Jellyfish</li><li>Seated Side Stretches and Twist</li><li>Supine Pranayama- 8-10 minutes.</li><li>*Turn lights down and offer blankets if the room temperature is cool.</li><li>*Have students turn off phones completely to experience an EMF free environment.</li><li>Instruct students to apply eye pillows, if it feels right.</li><li>Begin the practice with no music to cleanse their auditory channels.</li><li>Lie down on your back, preferably propping your torso up with a rolled-up mat or bolster and elevate your head with a blanket or sweatshirt. Let the arms drop to the sides and your legs extend out in front of you.</li><li>Begin to simply observe the breath, noticing its rhythms and pathways.</li><li>Now start to slow the breath down by breathing through the nostrils, observing sensations of the inhalation versus the exhalation at the nostrils.</li><li>Yogic breathing emphasizes nostril breathing to regulate the nervous system.</li><li>Feel the breath fill the collarbone region, with a gentle lifting and lowering.</li><li>Focus the breath at the chest, feeling the muscles of the chest expand and contract.</li><li>Finally, breathe into the ribs to initiate movement in the diaphragm and belly.</li><li>It takes time to relax the belly and let the breath drop deeply into the lungs.</li><li>Eventually you'll be able to expand the sides of the waist, the belly and even the lower back.</li><li>Continue with breathing guidance until they have the hang of it before letting them breathe independently.</li></ul>**Closing:**<ul><li>Savasana - Roll to one side to remove the props beneath you and rest on your mat. Relax the entire body from head to toe, through guided relaxation by the teacher.</li><li>Play soft, instrumental music.</li></ul>

Daily Lesson Plan #4:
Natural Breath

- Complete the breath practice by sitting up and have each student lift their feather to their face. Breathe in and out through the nostrils, the ideal way to breathe and watch the feather move with the breath. Just like wind, or sunlight, we can't touch our breath, but we can see and feel the effects of it.
- Suggested quote: "The practice of Yoga creates an inner relaxation that accompanies a peaceful state of being."

Reflection/Conclusion

- With music still playing, rise to sitting and inhale arms overhead, exhaling hands together, lowering to heart center. Do this three times to introduce the concept of moving with the breath. Now accompany the music and exhale to the sound of OM. OM or Aum, has four phases, A...U...M...Silence.
- Thank your classmates for sharing the experience by drawing hands to the heart center and saying "Namaste, the light in me honors the light in you."

OMwork

Find time between your Yoga classes to practice your natural breath, in any body shape (sitting, standing or lying down). Reflect and journal on insights or observations you have about your own unique and mostly unconscious breathing patterns.

OMwork Material

- Breathing Log

Breathing Log

For one week, reflect on any insights or observations you have about your unique breathing patterns.

Date & Time	
Type of Breath	
Situation	
Feeling at the Time	
What changes, if any, did you make to your breath?	
After the change or acknowledgement of breath, what did you notice?	

Daily Lesson Plan #5: Breathing Flow

Intention/Objective
To awaken the breath and coordinate it with movement.
Teaching Resource Material
<ul><li>Instruct students to retrieve a mat, block and band (a trauma-sensitive term for belt or strap) and then return them at the end of class. They will be expected to do this for each class.</li><li>Play soft, instrumental music and dim the lights.</li></ul>
Review/Introduction
<ul><li>Discuss observations about students' breathing patterns. We are breathing machines; it's what the body is designed to do but our lifestyle can impair this instinct.</li><li>Introduction to props: They are used for finding proper alignment, ensuring safety, avoiding injury and helping us glean the most benefit from the asana.</li><li>Mats: It provides a non-slip surface for hands and feet. Socks increase our risk of slipping and therefore, yoga is typically practiced in bare feet.</li><li>Note: Feet are a source of great angst, so many students will keep socks on. However, emphasize the importance of bare feet. We always want to make sure that the hands and feet are always on the same surface.</li><li>Bands (aka belts or straps): Used to connect hand to foot when the reach is not long enough, also used to train body parts to remain in proper alignment.</li><li>Blocks: These offer extra height and support when needed. There are three heights available with your block:<ul><li>Highest height: Papa Bear/Tadasana</li><li>Middle height: Mama Bear/Dandasana</li><li>Lowest height: Baby Bear/Savasana</li></ul></li><li>Chairs: Helpful for modifications and stabilization in balance forms.</li><li>Eye pillows: Used for restorative asanas to help draw senses inward and turn off external stimuli. Pressure of the pillow is also effective for relieving tension headaches.</li></ul>
Lesson
This asana sequence mainly targets the side waist, which needs to open if the lungs are to breathe deeply and fully absorb oxygen. The deepest benefits of asanas occur when the side waist participates in lengthening. **Centering:**<ul><li>Seated side stretch, sit cross legged in Sukhasana and reach right arm overhead. Find out how deeply you can breathe into your right side. Strong, deep, smooth breathing. Rise and switch leg position, then reach overhead with your left arm. Fill every air sac in the lungs with breath and energy.</li></ul>**Body of Class:**<ul><li>Mountain/Tadasana</li><li>Standing Half Moon Side Stretch/aka Banana</li><li>The Monkey: In Mountain, step feet mat width apart and make fists with your hands. Inhale with the torso centered and exhale while leaning to the left, sliding the left hand down the leg while the right fist tucks into the right armpit. Inhale back to center and exhale to the other side. Pick up speed to warm up the body and transition into saying "Ha" on the exhalations to increase power.</li><li>Lunge with blocks on each side of the front foot for hands to rest on. Right side first, then left side.</li></ul>

- Lunge again with hands on blocks, then rise to Crescent Lunge (arms reaching overhead). Right side first, then switch to the left. Flow with your breath.
- Downward Dog to Plank to Table, sweep lower legs to right and open to Side Plank/Vasisthasana on right knee and hand, with upper arm reaching diagonally. Both sides. Flow with your breath.
- Child's (five breaths or more), then inhale up to plank on knees, lower to Chaturanga on knees and return to Child's. 3x.
- Same sequence above but add Cobra, so from Child's rise to plank on knees, to Chaturanga to Cobra and return to Child's, 3x. Flow with your breath.
- Downward Dog with five exhalations with a "Ha" to disperse stress, then step or jump through to sitting.
- Staff/Dandasana
- Head to Knee/Janu Sirsasana, flow with your breath.

Closing:
- Partner Asana: Bound Angle/Baddha Konasana. Back-to-back, one partner leans back with their feet on the mat, pressing on the spine while the other folds forward into Baddha Konasana.
- Savasana with eye pillow - let the wisdom of the breath find its own rhythm inside your body.

Reflection/Conclusion

Partner work:
- In partners or in small groups, discuss how you feel and any challenges you encountered (such as drowsiness, mental distraction, nausea).
- Thank your classmates with Namaste and as a class, share any closing remarks on how you feel and how you're breathing.

OMwork

Research three definitions of Namaste and note your favorite one.

OMwork Material

Namaste Definition Omwork

Namaste Definition

Curriculum Outcomes

- Students will apply their understanding of yogic principles to their yoga practice.
- Students will explore relaxation techniques for quieting thoughts and managing emotions and stress.
- Students will identify the techniques that are most effective for them.
- Students will apply the principles of yoga in a personal way outside of yoga practice.

Research the three possible definitions of Namaste. State your favourite one and explain why.

Daily Lesson Plan #6: Namaste

Intention/Objective
Identify the powerful message within the special term Namaste and apply it to life and practice.
Teaching Resource Material
Craft paper, scissors, crayons, markers etc.
Review/Introduction
In partners, Partner A relaxes on their back while Partner B takes two minutes to talk Partner A through the process of finding their natural breath. Switch roles.
Lesson

Centering:
- Let's consider that we are pure beings having an imperfect human experience and that we all share the same breath.
- Stir the Pot: Sitting in Easy or Friendship Asana (on a chair), begin to circle the torso over the pelvis in one direction, then the other. Imagine a pencil at the top of the head initially drawing small circles, then larger ones, and back to small ones.
- Seated Side Stretch
- Rising to Mountain, inhale and reach arms overhead and exhale hands to the heart.
- Lower into modified or full Yogic Squat/Malasana. Take a breath here and then exhale, lift the hips, hang the head. Inhale curl back up to standing, arms reaching and repeat 10x to warm up the legs, hips and lower back.

Body of Class:
- Mountain to Powerful/Utkatasana to Standing forward fold/Padangusthasana back to Mountain, 3x, sinking deeper each round.
- Sun Breaths 3x.
- As you rise to Extended Mountain, explore with your eye gaze, by first lifting the head and then the eyes, and then lead with the eyes and then the head. This showcases how our eye gaze-Drishti influences each asana.
- From Mountain, step back to Table and lift the right leg, followed by the left for five breaths each.
- Downward Dog
- Extend the right leg up and back into a three-legged dog for five breaths and lower. Do the same on the left.
- Release to Child's/Balasana for five breaths, then reach to the right side for five breaths and to the left for five breaths.

Closing:
- Lift torso and take a moment in Cross Legged/Sukhasana to center oneself.
- Come to sit in a circle and discuss the students' research on Namaste and collectively decide upon a phrase that they will use to close the class, such as "The light in me honors the light in you."
- Students can draw and cut out the word Namaste with hands at heart symbol and the agreed upon description and present it on the wall.
- Savasana, with a song, like "I am Not My Hair", by India Arie or "Scars to Your Beautiful", by Alessia Cara

Reflection/Conclusion
Turn to two people in your class, make direct eye contact, if your culture allows, and repeat the Namaste definition to one another.

Daily Lesson Plan #6:
Namaste

OMwork
• Read the handout on the Koshas and report on the correlation between the Koshas and namaste. • Research Drishti and explain in a one-page essay, double spaced, its importance during asana practice and in our lives.
OMwork Material
Koshas - The Layers of the Self Handout

Koshas – The Layers of the Self

Many people spend hundreds—sometimes thousands—of dollars each year enhancing their outward appearance, from manicures and lash extensions to designer clothing. Personal adornment and hygiene have been part of human life for centuries, often reflecting self-respect and creative expression. However, in today's culture, this focus has become excessive, leading to an unhealthy obsession with physical appearance. It's important to remember that who we are goes far beyond what we look like.

Yoga teaches that we are made up of multiple layers, or aspects, that make us human. Interestingly, the physical body—the one we tend to focus on the most—is actually the outermost and most superficial of these layers, furthest from our true essence.

To help understand this, imagine a lightbulb covered by several lampshades. You, the true Self, are the bulb—the source of light. The lampshades represent layers that soften and obscure that light to varying degrees. These layers are known in yoga as the *koshas*, or "sheaths" of being.

Annamaya Kosha

The first and most external sheath is the *Annamaya Kosha*, also called the "food body." This is the physical body, experienced through the five senses and shaped by what we consume. The ancient saying, "You are what you eat," rings true here—yogis believed that the food and substances we take in become the very cells of our body.

Everything in the material world—including our physical form—goes through constant change, eventually returning to the earth. For this reason, the *Annamaya Kosha* is marked by impermanence. Through the practice of *asanas* (yoga postures), we care for and strengthen this layer, preparing ourselves to turn inward and connect with the deeper, more enduring aspects of who we are.

Pranamaya Kosha

The second layer of our being is the *Pranamaya Kosha*, or energy body. This subtle field of energy gives us vitality—it's what fuels our movement, passion, and ability to pursue dreams and visions. Unlike the thinking mind, this layer is felt through sensation and intuition.

Though invisible, our energy body is deeply affected by what we eat, the music we listen to, the quality of our relationships, our environment, and our activity levels. Despite its subtle nature, it has a profound impact on our physical health and emotional well-being.

We can nourish both the physical and energetic bodies by drinking clean water, eating nutrient-rich foods, spending time in sunlight and fresh air, and engaging in loving, peaceful interactions with people and pets. On the other hand, our energy can be depleted by stress, poor posture, excessive screen time, and lack of movement.

Through yoga postures (*asanas*) and breath control (*pranayama*), we learn to regulate and refine this energetic layer, helping us shift our focus inward, toward the deeper layers of the self.

Manomaya and Vijnanamaya Koshas

The next two *koshas* belong to what's known as the "subtle body." They are the *Manomaya Kosha*, the mental body, and the *Vijnanamaya Kosha*, the wisdom body.

The *Manomaya Kosha* governs our thoughts, beliefs, emotions, and sensory impressions—essentially the processes of the thinking mind. The *Vijnanamaya Kosha*, by contrast, is the inner wisdom layer, home to our discernment and intuitive understanding of truth.

In modern culture, we are often encouraged to stop here, over-identifying with intellect and academic success. But when we remain stuck in the mind, disconnected from deeper awareness, it can lead to a lack of meaning, purpose, and authentic connection.

Through yoga and mindfulness, we begin to calm the busy, reactive mind and access the higher wisdom of the *Vijnanamaya Kosha*. This shift brings clarity, insight, and a deeper understanding of our true nature.

Anandamaya Kosha

At the core of our being is the *Anandamaya Kosha*—the bliss body. This is not fleeting happiness that depends on external circumstances, but a deep, abiding joy, peace, and love that arises from within. Here, we feel at home, grounded in a spacious, unified awareness that transcends the fluctuations of the outer world.

This innermost layer is where we experience our purest state of being. It is our essence, our light—the radiance that shines through all the other layers.

When we say *Namaste* at the end of a yoga class, we are acknowledging this light in one another. We look beyond the surface—beyond physical form, thoughts, and emotions—and honour the divine presence within each of us.

Through continued practice—yoga, mindfulness, and other contemplative traditions—we slowly loosen our grip on the need for external perfection. In doing so, we reconnect with the enduring light of our true self.

Daily Lesson Plan #7: Mountain Introduction

Intention/Objective
Students will gain understanding of: <ul><li>Proper postural alignment</li><li>The detriment of poor posture</li><li>The lasting benefits of body alignment</li></ul>
Teaching Resource Material
<ul><li>Tadasana/Samasthiti Benefits and Teaching Points</li><li>Tadasana Peer Evaluation</li></ul>
Review/Introduction
<ul><li>In groups of four or five, invite each group to create the word yoga with their bodies. Keep the instruction minimal so they can exercise their own creativity.</li><li>Koshas- while in their small groups, have students create a body shape that demonstrates the koshas and the luminous light within.</li><li>The first and most important asana is Mountain/Tadasana/Samastithi. It is the most important asana because every other asana includes the alignment details of Mountain.</li></ul>
Lesson
Mountain Affirmation: "I fill out my body with confidence, kindness and relaxed awareness." <ul><li>Throughout the practice repeat this, or similar affirmations that support the mindset of Mountain.</li><li>Anatomy: Introduce the spine and the axial skeleton, see YTT anatomy sessions for more details.</li></ul> **Centering:** <ul><li>Students can take photos of their partners standing posture BEFORE Mountain instructions.</li><li>Neck stretches</li><li>Sun Breaths three times</li><li>Standing Half Moon (AKA Banana in Yoga Posters-Level 1).</li></ul> **Body of Class:** <ul><li>Mountain against the wall:</li><li>Stand with heels three inches from the wall</li><li>Press tailbone, shoulder blades and head against the wall (the kyphotic curves)</li><li>Can you press the outer back portion of the shoulders toward the wall?</li><li>Slide a hand between the wall and the lower back to ensure the lumbar curve exists and between the wall and the neck to ensure proper cervical curve (these are lordotic curves).</li></ul> **Question:** <ul><li>Why does the spine have curves? (to absorb compression)</li><li>With these three points of contact, give your full attention to your posture and breathing and step away from the wall. Walk around the room, noticing how natural or foreign this alignment feels.</li><li>Try to relax the neck and breathe as you retrain your spine to stand and walk with proper alignment.</li></ul> **Mountain partner exercise:** <ul><li>Using the student handout on Mountain, have them coach each other through Mountain by standing beside their partner and making suggestions for better alignment.</li><li>Take a second photo of your partner in Mountain.</li></ul> **Closing:**   Savasana, guiding students through the koshic layers of the self.
Reflection/Conclusion

Daily Lesson Plan #7:
Mountain Introduction

Students can rise to standing and read the affirmation for Mountain in unison: "I fill out my body with confidence, kindness and relaxed awareness."
OMwork
<ul><li>Journal about your new asana, Mountain, and how you feel in this stance. Note the differences between the photo of you at the beginning and your alignment after Mountain instruction.</li><li>Answer these two questions:</li><li>What muscles need to be strengthened?</li><li>What muscles need to be stretched?</li><li>Letter to self: Write a letter to yourself addressing the reasons why you registered for this course, what it is you wish to accomplish in the next four months and how do you want to feel by the end of it. This is to be submitted and then added to your wellness portfolio.</li></ul>
OMwork Material
Mountain Benefits handout Mountain Teaching Points Mountain Peer Evaluation

Mountain – Tadasana / Samasthiti Benefits of Practicing Proper Posture

- Promotes optimal spinal alignment, improving blood circulation throughout the body
- Encourages proper standing posture, helping to prevent joint stress caused by uneven weight distribution
- Tones the pelvic floor and strengthens core abdominal muscles
- Builds strength in the arches of the feet, as well as the knees, legs, and back
- Expands lung capacity by supporting deep, full breathing
- Enhances mental focus, clarity, and present-moment awareness
- Boosts self-confidence and cultivates a sense of inner strength
- May improve interpersonal relationships and contribute to career success by enhancing presence and posture
- Helps alleviate mild symptoms of anxiety and depression
- Supports healthy digestion through gentle abdominal engagement and improved alignment
- Aids in the prevention of osteoarthritis by encouraging balanced joint function and muscle engagement

Mountain – Tadasana / Samasthiti

Teaching Points Using the ACE Principle (Anchor, Core, Expression)

Optional Pre-Activity

Have students take photos of each other in their natural standing posture before alignment instruction. This helps them observe their habitual stance and track progress.

Anchor – Grounding & Stability

- Bring the mounds of the big toes together or stand with feet hip-width apart for comfort and stability.

- Turn the feet to point straight forward, allowing the heels to be slightly apart.
- Lift the toes, spread them wide (spacious "yogi toes"), then slowly lower them down.
- Ground evenly through the **three points** of each foot:
  - Mound of the big toe
  - Mound of the pinky toe
  - Center of the heel
- Lift the arches of the feet.
- Engage the quadriceps (front thighs) to stabilize the legs.

Core – Integrity & Internal Support

- Engage the **pelvic floor** (as if you were gently holding in urine).
- Find **neutral pelvis** by lengthening the 'tail' bone down toward the earth.
- Engage **Uddiyana Bandha** by exhaling and drawing the lower belly back toward the spine (without holding the breath).
- Activate **Empowered Breathing**:
  - Inhale to expand and lengthen the trunk
  - Maintain the lift of the ribcage on the exhalation
- Feel your torso supported and uplifted from within.

Expression – Extension & Energetic Expansion

- Arms extend straight, with fingers actively reaching toward the outer ankles.
- Lift the **sternum** (breastbone) without flaring the ribs.
- Gently tuck the bottom tips of the shoulder blades into the back body.
- Keep the **chin parallel to the floor**, head stacked directly above the spine.
- **Lift through the crown of the head**, elongating the spine.
- Feel the dual action of:
  - **Grounding from the waist down** like the roots of a tree
  - **Expanding from the waist up** like branches reaching toward the sky

Final Alignment Check – "The Plum Line"

- Ears, shoulders, hips, and ankles should stack in a straight line when viewed from the side.
- Consider using a string with a small weight (a "plumb line") as a visual aid to demonstrate this vertical alignment.

Daily Lesson Plan #7:
Mountain Introduction

Mountain / Tadasana – Peer Evaluation

Group Activity Instructions

In groups of **three**, rotate through each of the following roles:
- **Partner 1 – Teacher**: Lead one group member through the key teaching points of Tadasana.
- **Partner 2 – Student**: Follow the teacher's verbal instructions and adjust your posture.
- **Partner 3 – Evaluator**:
    - Take a **photo** of the student in their **natural stance** before alignment.
    - Check off the teaching points the teacher includes.
    - Take a **photo** of the student in **Tadasana**, to compare "before and after" alignment.

Teacher Name: _____

Evaluator Name: _____

Teaching Points Checklist for Tadasana

Check off each point as the teacher cues or explains it:
- ☐ Begin standing with feet together, or hip-width apart.
- ☐ Ground down through the **tripod** of each foot (big toe mound, pinky toe mound, heel).
- ☐ Lift arches and toes; **spread toes** wide and softly lower them.
- ☐ Engage the **quadriceps/front thighs** by lifting the kneecaps.
- ☐ Drop the tailbone and find **neutral pelvis**.
- ☐ Engage **Uddiyana Bandha** by exhaling and drawing lower belly toward spine.
- ☐ Emphasize **Empowered (diaphragmatic) breathing**.
- ☐ Lift the **sternum** (breastbone).
- ☐ **Tuck shoulder blades** gently into the back ribs.
- ☐ Chin is **parallel to the floor**.
- ☐ Head draws slightly back, stacking over the spine.
- ☐ Lengthen upward through the **crown of the head**.
- ☐ From the waist down: **ground into the earth** like tree roots.
- ☐ From the waist up: **rise and expand** like tree branches.
- ☐ Check vertical alignment: **ears → shoulders → hips → ankles**.
- ☐ Recite or invite the affirmation:

"I fill out my body with confidence, kindness, and relaxed awareness."

Daily Lesson Plan #8: Mountain in Motion

Intention/Objective
Students will apply their understanding of proper postural alignment to other asanas. *Plumb lines can be available for students to explore while students are arriving or leaving class. One partner reaches up to hold the plum line while the other stands beside the plum line. Your partner can serve as your mirror to help direct your movements to find alignment.
Teaching Resource Materials
Class sets of three-foot-long dowels or Plumb Lines (a long string with stone tied at the bottom)
Review/Introduction
Begin the class by having students instruct you through the mechanics of Mountain. Encourage them to start at the feet and instruct upward, to the core and then extension, emphasizing the importance of laying the foundation of every asana first.
Lesson

Centering:
- In Sukhasana or Virasana, reconnect with your natural breath, soften your belly while keeping the spine tall. Can you relax your gaze (drishti) and your jaw while breathing through the nostrils?
- This is like cleaning the slate, clearing the body of existing tension, holding patterns that cause weakness. Draw awareness to the length and alignment of your spine, teaching the body how to find proper alignment of Mountain in a seated position.
- For Supine Mountain, lay down and bring your arms alongside the torso, palms facing the thighs. Reach the fingertips to the outer ankles. Press heels away and draw toes toward the face, activating the legs. Gently press the belly button into the floor and reach the tailbone to the heels. Slide shoulder blades down the back and tuck the chin while lifting the base of the skull away from the neck. This is Supine Mountain (Supta Samasthiti). Notice the three aspects of the spine in contact with the floor-tailbone, mid-back and head. This indicates the S curve in our spines, with arches at the lower back and neck, which absorb compression.

Body of Class:
- Leg lifts ten times. This exercise awakens the deep core channels of the inner thighs and pelvic floor, necessary for a strong Mountain form.
- On your back, place a block between thighs and interlock fingers behind the head. Lift the legs straight up and squeeze the block as you exhale. At the same time, lift the head, drawing your elbows and nose toward the thighs without straining the neck. Inhale and release the head down and lower the legs. Exhale as you lift legs and head; inhale as you lower. Gradually add a lift in the tailbone as the head lifts to engage the deep core muscles. **Caution:** Watch that students do not strain their necks.
- Plankasana on elbows with a block between thighs for 30 seconds, three times.
- Remove the block, tuck knees to chest and rock and roll a few times, gradually rolling up to sitting, and back onto the shoulders. Keep rocking forward and back to gradually gain momentum to rise to sitting or even standing (or rise in their own way).
- When standing, come to the top of your mat and plant your feet together or hip width apart.
- Neck stretches
- Standing Half Moon/Banana/Standing Ardha Chandrasana

Daily Lesson Plan #8:
Mountain in Motion

- Anahatasana - a heart opener with fingers interlaced behind the back in Yoga Mudra. Inhale and lift arms up away from the backside
- Yoga Mudra - with fingers interlaced behind, exhale fold forward, letting the arms release away from the backside. Inhale rise back up and repeat one more time, switching hand positions to break habitual patterns that cause imbalances in the body and mind.
- Chest stretches: Stand with your right side along the wall and reach the right arm back, palm against wall. With your left hand on the wall in front of the chest, press your torso toward the center of the room, stretching through the right chest and biceps - common muscle groups that shorten and tighten from slouching or desk work.
- Mountain: Revisit Resource Material
- Mountain Affirmation: "I fill out my body with confidence, kindness and relaxed awareness."
- Don't forget to smile!
- Sun Salutation Prep: Flow from Tadasana to Urdhva Hastasana (extended Mountain) to Downward Dog to Plank to Chaturanga (knees dropped initially), back to Downward dog to Mountain pose. Can you find Mountain in each of these postures?
- Partner work: Using a dowel, stand beside your partner as the teacher guides students through the flow sequence. Take five breaths in each asana to offer time for the partner to place the dowel along the person's spine to check for Mountain alignment. Switch roles so the teacher can instruct the next group.

Closing:
- Supine Twist/Jathara Parivartanasana
- Relaxation/Savasana
- Reflection: find comfort here, resting in the belief that you are a good and infinitely capable person.

Reflection/Conclusion
By asking the body to shift and grow, it is important to keep our minds open to healthier ways of being in the world as well. Has anyone in your life noticed changes in you already?

OMwork

Anatomy Assignment:
After exploring Mountain, assess your own standing posture and record areas of weakness (overstretched muscles) and areas of tension (short muscles). How might you improve your stance? Place findings in your wellness portfolio.

OMwork Material
- Posture Alignment Rubric
- Mountain Reflection

Posture Alignment Rubric

Throughout the day, our mood, energy, and breath can shift—sometimes dramatically—and these changes often show up in our posture. Over the next week, observe your standing alignment and how it reflects your inner state.

Instructions:
- Complete the chart twice daily:
    - Morning (beginning of the school day)
    - Afternoon (end of the school day)
- Make short notes about:
    - Your **physical posture**
    - How your **body feels**
    - Your **mental/emotional state**
    - The **quality of your breath**

Daily Lesson Plan #8:
Mountain in Motion

Curriculum Outcomes

Demonstrate foundational asanas with proper alignment
Develop awareness of the mind–body connection

Posture Observation Chart

Date	
Time	
How is my posture?	
Activity	
Postural Adjustment	

Mountain Reflection

Take a few moments to reflect on your experience with posture and alignment this week. Use the questions below as a guide. Be honest and thoughtful—this journal is for you to better understand your body, mind, and habits.

Journal Prompts

1. **Awareness:** Did this exercise make you more aware of your standing alignment than you normally would be? How so?
2. **Ongoing Attention:** Do you think you'll continue to pay attention to your posture regularly? Why or why not?
3. **Self-Assessment:** What did you notice are the strengths of your posture? What about your areas for improvement?
4. **Impact of the Assignment:** Based on this assignment, how do you think your posture will change going forward?
5. **Mind–Body Connection:** Did you notice any relationship between the time of day, your mood, or energy level, and the way you were standing? Explain your observations.
6. **Personal Discovery:** After reviewing your posture data from the week, what did you discover about your alignment?

Closing Reflection

Stand tall in this body of yours, and you turn your feet in the direction of your true path.
   Take a deep breath. Acknowledge the work you've done.
   You're learning to stand not just with your body, but with intention.

Daily Lesson Plan #9:
Mountain Mindfulness Practice

Script for Teacher to Read

Begin by finding a comfortable seated position.

Prop your hips up on a block or a rolled-up edge of your yoga mat. You may choose to rest your back gently against a wall for additional support.

Place your hands on your thighs, forming Jnana Mudra by touching the tips of your thumbs and index fingers together.

Roll your shoulders up and back, allowing the shoulder blades to feel heavy.

Tuck your chin slightly to align your ears over your shoulders.

Imagine your spine as a tower of building blocks—adjust your posture so that each "block" supports the next, creating a strong, stable foundation.

Now, begin to notice your breath.

Feel the air as it enters your nose, expanding your collarbones and chest.

Let your breath travel deep into your belly—allowing it to gently rise and fall.

Inhale slowly and deeply. Exhale fully and completely.

As your breath becomes steady, begin to imagine your body becoming a mountain.

Your seat is the solid granite base, rooted deep into the earth.

The crown of your head becomes the mountain's peak, rising into the sky.

Now, picture the life that moves across the surface of your mountain—

Birds fly overhead, animals move freely, and wildflowers bloom.

But beneath all this activity, the *mountain remains unchanged.*

It is steady, grounded, and deeply connected to the earth.

As time passes, the days grow shorter and the air becomes cooler.

Leaves transform into brilliant shades of orange, red, and gold.

Still, the mountain stays the same—strong, grounded, and untouched by the change above.

Autumn fades. Winds blow stronger.

Leaves fall, one by one—until only a single leaf remains.

With one final gust, it is lifted into the air, floating freely.

This reminds us: letting go is part of nature's rhythm.

And even in letting go, the mountain stands firm.

Winter comes.

Snowflakes fall gently at first, then whip across the mountain's face.

Winds howl, ice forms—but the core of the mountain remains unmoved, still anchored deep into the earth.

Eventually, the days grow longer.

The snow and ice begin to melt.

Once again, the surface of the mountain is revealed.

From beneath the soil, new life emerges—first a sprout, then many.

Buds bloom. Flowers open. Colors return.

Animals move freely again. The surface changes, yet the mountain remains as it always was: grounded, stable, whole.

Daily Lesson Plan #9:
Mountain Mindfulness Practice

Just like the mountain, *you* experience seasons—
Sometimes within a day, even within a single moment.
Emotions come and go. External circumstances shift.
But beneath it all, *you are the mountain.*
You are rooted.
You are steady.
You are enough.
Begin to bring gentle movement to your fingers and toes.
If you've been lying down, slowly rise to sit.
Come to standing, placing your feet hip-width apart.
Find Tadasana/Mountain.
Let your body rise tall, rooted through your feet, lifted through your crown.

Ask yourself

- How do I feel in this moment?
- Is this sensation new or different?
- How might this awareness shift my thoughts and actions when I encounter life's challenges?

Follow-Up Suggestions

- If time allows guide students through a few gentle **Sun Salutations (Namaskars)** while encouraging them to maintain this sense of grounded awareness.
- Conclude class with quiet reflection time. Invite students to complete a short writing assignment or journal entry based on the meditation.

Student Reflection Questions

1. How do I feel now after practicing the Mountain Practice?
2. How will this awareness help me respond to stress or overwhelm in the future?
3. What stood out most to me during this visualization?

Encourage students to add any personal insights or reflections that arose during their experience.

Daily Lesson Plan #10:
Sun Salutation A/Surya Namaskar A

Intention/Objective
Introduce Surya Namaskar while applying the principles of Mountain.
Teaching Resource Material
Sun Breath and Sun Salutation A Scripts
Review/Introduction
<ul><li>Have the following affirmation displayed on the board or on an overhead: Sun Salutation Affirmation:" I salute the radiant sun, and the awakening light within".</li><li>Guide students to unleash their Natural Breath, followed by Empowered Diaphragmatic Breathing in preparation for Vinyasa (movement coordinated with breath).</li><li>Empowered Breathing focuses on the diaphragm, the main breathing muscles, keeping the breath at the rib cage, instead of dropping into the belly, which can disperse our energy during movement.</li></ul>
Lesson
Core Cultivation:<ul><li>Explain the anatomy of core engagement in the trunk, from Mula Bandha to Uddiyana to the obliques, to the spinal muscles. Have them engage the muscle groups as they are explained.</li></ul>**Centering:**<ul><li>Sukhasana to Jellyfish, working the Bandhas: find a comfortable seat and lift the ribs, engaging the pelvic floor by pulling up through the central pelvic muscles. Now inhale and arch the spine, slightly looking up and exhale, round the back, curling the head toward your navel. Continue this movement for about 10-12 cycles.</li><li>As you inhale, engage the spinal muscles.</li><li>As you exhale, pull the belly back toward the spine so this becomes a core cultivation exercise.</li><li>By awakening the spine, through flexion and extension, we activate Mula and Uddiyana Bandhas, and release tension in the diaphragm, the main breathing muscle in the body.</li><li>Sun Breaths: Read from script</li><li>Through the full spectrum of movement, the spine remains long and the core strong as the body folds and rises. If the legs need to bend to accommodate for tension, that's fine at this stage.</li><li>Flow through 3 more Sun Breaths, learning to keep core muscles alive while breathing in concert with the movements. This is called Vinyasa, moving in coordination with your breath.</li></ul>**Body of Class:**<ul><li>Introduce Sun Salutation A by demonstrating the basic version first, (walking vs. jumping, dropping to knees and doing Cobra vs. Upward Facing Dog) then have students join in for two slow salutations altogether.</li><li>For the next one, the teacher can wander around the room, encouraging Mountain throughout the sequence (except in Cobra). This will build strength in postural muscles (along the spine and core), helping students to stand tall with less effort.</li><li>Teacher can workshop any misalignments noticed throughout the Namaskar (like dropping the head first in Chaturanga) and clarify any questions about breathing or sequencing.</li><li>*Teaching Tip- watch for rounding of the mid back in Ardha Uttanasana/long spine. Many will round the spine to accommodate for tight hamstrings so instruct them to bend the knees and squeeze the shoulder blades together, keeping the neck long.</li></ul>

Closing: • Explain that building heat is the goal for Sun Salutations (solar energy) and for our asana practice at large. Heat helps to warm up the body, cleanse toxins and burn excess body fat. • Knees to chest/Apanasana with a contraction of every muscle and then to a count of 15 slowly extend the legs and rest on your back. • Savasana with soft instrumental music.
Reflection/Conclusion
Thank your classmates for the journey, closing with Namaste.
OMwork

• Suggested reading: *E.g., Health Benefits of Sun Salutations*
• Practice assignment: *Complete 5 rounds of Surya Namaskar A with breath holds in Downward Dog*
• Journaling prompts:
  1. How did you feel before and after your personal practice?
  2. What physical or emotional shifts did you notice?
  3. Any insights about breath, posture, or energy?

OMwork Material
• Health Benefits of the Sun Salutations • Sun Breath and Sun Salutation A Scripts

Surya Namaskar: The Complete Practice

Surya Namaskar (Sun Salutation) delivers all the core benefits of yoga in a single, accessible practice. This warming sequence strengthens and awakens the body, sharpens mental clarity, and supports emotional balance. It:
- Challenges major muscle groups
- Lubricates joints and ligaments
- Improves posture, flexibility, and balance

Beyond these physical gains, Surya Namaskar conditions every internal system of the body:
- **Cardiovascular system:** Oxygenates the blood, improving heart health
- **Digestive system:** Stimulates metabolism and improves organ function
- **Lymphatic system:** Enhances detoxification and immune support
- **Respiratory system:** Controlled breathing deepens lung capacity
- **Nervous system:** Induces calm and supports stress relief
- **Endocrine system:** Balances hormones—especially helpful for teens!

By triggering the relaxation response, this practice helps relieve tension, stress, and anxiety, often linked to poor breathing habits. As an energizing alternative to caffeine or stimulants, it may also support more restful sleep over time.

Energy of Sun Salutations

In yogic philosophy, prana is our life-force energy, flowing through nadis, or energy channels (similar to meridians in Traditional Chinese Medicine). There are said to be over 72,000 nadis in the body, with three primary pathways:
- **Ida Nadi** – begins on the left side; governs cooling, lunar energy
- **Pingala Nadi** – begins on the right side; governs heating, solar energy
- **Sushumna Nadi** – the central channel, running up the spine to the crown of the head

Yoga asanas—especially flowing sequences like Surya Namaskar—help open and unblock these pathways, allowing prana to move freely. When energy flows well, we feel:
- Inspired
- Creative
- Grounded
- Harmonious

When stress, tension, or stagnation occur (such as tightness in the neck or shoulders), prana cannot circulate properly. This can result in physical symptoms like headaches or chronic pain. Over time, lack of circulation can lead to "dis-ease." Yoga helps reverse this, restoring balance, vitality, and ease throughout the body.

Sun Breath & Sun Salutation A/Surya Namaskar A Scripts

Teaching tip: We generally inhale when we open or increase the angle of the body and exhale when we close or decrease the angle of the body.

Ancient Wisdom, Modern Relevance

Most yoga postures are named after animals, inspired by yogis who observed the natural healing behaviors of animals in the wild. For instance, Cobra (Bhujangasana), mimics a snake arching its back to energize and stimulate the spine.

Surya Namaskar, originally performed to greet the rising sun, honors the Sun Teacher—the ancient guide of illumination. Today, scientific research supports what yogis long understood: morning sunlight regulates our circadian rhythms and supports overall wellness.

Sun Salutations awaken the body by:
- Activating all major muscle groups
- Linking movement with rhythmic breath
- Creating internal heat to stimulate detoxification

This flowing sequence truly embodies yoga's ability to connect mind, body, breath, and spirit—energizing your day from the inside out.

Sun Breath Script:

- Begin in Mountain
- Inhale arms up to Extended Mountain
- Exhale hinge at the hips and fold
- Inhale to a flat back
- Exhale fold again
- Inhale rise to Extended Mountain
- Exhale to Mountain

Modified Sun Salutation/Surya Namaskar A Script:

Sun Salutation Affirmation: I salute the Sun, and the awakening light within.

- Mountain
- Inhale arms up to extended Mountain
- Exhale hinge into a forward fold
- Inhale to a flat back
- Exhale to Plankasana on knees, and take a few breaths
- Exhale lower body to the floor
- Inhale rise to Cobra
- Exhale to tabletop or to Downward Facing Dog.
- Take Five breaths here in Downward Facing Dog, Table or Child's
- Inhale walk to the top of your mat and rise to flat back
- Exhale fold forward
- Inhale up to Extended Mountain
- Exhale to Mountain

Complete Sun Salutation/Surya Namaskar A Script

*It takes time to build strength and stamina, but like anything, practice makes progress.

*Spend some time on the transitions so they understand how to flow and breathe, before instructing with the traditional speed of half a breath per asana.

- Stand in Mountain and begin ujjayi breathing
- Inhale arms overhead to extended Mountain
- Exhale fold forward
- Inhale to a flat back
- Exhale step or jump back to Low Plank/Chaturanga Dandasana
- Inhale to Upward Facing Dog
- Exhale into Downward Dog for five breaths
- Inhale jump forward and rise to a flat back
- Exhale fold forward
- Inhale rise to Extended Mountain
- Exhale into Mountain

Note: Depending on the maturity (and history of trauma) of your group, you may wish to change the name of the downward dog to the Upside-Down V.

Daily Lesson Plan #11: Sun Salutation B/Surya Namaskar B

Intention/Objective
Students will apply their understanding of the Sun Breaths and Sun Salutations by practice teaching and progress to the practice of Sun Salutation B.
Teaching Resource Materials
Sun Salutation B Script
Review/Introduction
<ul><li>**Begin by reviewing the previous class and inviting students to share any questions or reflections about how they felt after practicing Sun Salutations.** Encourage them to notice and name where they feel sensation, tightness, or soreness in their bodies. Use this as an opportunity to introduce basic anatomical terms, helping them build body awareness and a shared vocabulary.</li><li>**Revisit the benefits of Sun Salutations**, emphasizing their role in generating internal heat—*tapas*—which warms the body, supports deeper stretching, and aids in detoxification.</li><li>**Facilitate a conversation about the various ways toxins enter our bodies**, such as through fast food, packaged or preserved items, polluted water and air, vaping, alcohol, and more. Explain how the accumulation of toxins over time can burden the body's systems and potentially contribute to conditions like allergies, autoimmune disorders, asthma, and even cancer.</li><li>**Make the connection between yoga and internal hygiene.** Just as we prioritize brushing our teeth or taking a daily shower, we can also care for our internal systems. Yoga offers tools for this kind of inner cleansing and renewal.</li><li>**Conclude by framing the practice as part of a larger lifestyle of self-care and intentional living.** This lays the foundation for understanding and embodying the *Yamas* and *Niyamas*, the ethical and personal observances that guide a yogic life.</li></ul>
Lesson
Centering:<ul><li>Begin in Mountain and with hands at heart, invite students to formulate an intention for their time on their mats today. Inhale arms overhead, palms touch, and exhale arms sweep down alongside the torso. Do this three times to review the concept of Vinyasa - simply coordinating breath and movement.</li><li>Have two or three students teach a Sun Breath, with the script on a wall or on a handout, attempting to cue the breath with the movement sequence. Be mindful of your language, using positive, encouraging words versus depreciating or humiliating language (revisiting the Yoga Class Agreement if need be).</li></ul>**Body of Class:**<ul><li>Sun Salutation A, three times</li><li>Refresh Uddiyana Bandha by placing first two fingers on the hip bones and slide them in two inches toward the centre of the belly. Draw the abdominals away from your fingers to awaken your transversus abdominis (the cummerbund or girdle of our abs) which is so important to protect the lumbar spine when doing Upward Dog.</li><li>With the core engaged, remind students of Empowered Breathing and speak to the significance of charging the torso with the breath instead of dropping it into the lower belly, which can diminish core stability.</li><li>Introduce Sun Salutation B with the accompanying script.</li><li>Analyze Powerful/Utkatasana and Warrior1/Virabhadrasana 1 by offering three or four key points only. Utkatasana can be taught facing the wall with fingertips on the wall in front,</li></ul>

lowering the hips while keeping the torso tall. It can also be taught with a wall squat, lowering hips level to knees to awaken the thighs.
- Explain what heel to heel alignment means for Warrior 1/Virabhadrasana 1. Proper positioning of the feet will allow the hip flexors to stretch, which are generally so tight due to chronic sitting.
- Neck caution- Remind them to maintain length in the neck as they tip the head back to look up at the thumbs.
- Bring it all together and do three Sun Salutation B's, attempting to keep the breath steady and deep.

Partner Form:
- Assisted Downward Dog - this introduces the concept of assists and respectful teamwork.
- Step on each side of your partner's hands while they are in downward dog, facing your partner's hips and press the heel of the palms into the crest of the hips to draw the tailbone up and away.
- Partner Downward Dog: The assistant turns so their feet are in the same direction as the student's hands in downward dog. The assistant places his/her hands in front of the partners hands and places the arches of the feet along their partner's hip crests and pushes their hips upward and away from the hands. This could be extended into a group downward dog form, with the strongest student at the back.

Closing:
- In Easy Asana/Sukhasana or Friendship/Maitryasana, find Yoga Mudra, by taking one wrist with the other hand behind the torso and fold forward on the exhalation, bowing to all that is good within you. Inhale up and exhale down three times then switch legs and hand positioning and do it on the other side three times. Do this to seal the benefits of the practice in the body/mind.
- Savasana

Reflection/Conclusion
Observe your body's sensations and any uplifting side effects that your practice has had on your attitude.

OMwork
Practice Sun Salutation A and B first thing in the morning and record observations in your journal.

OMwork Material
- Sun Salutation B Script
- Namaskar Project and Rubric Handouts

Surya Namaskar B – Sun Salutation B Script

Affirmation

"I salute the Sun and the awakening light within. I connect to my inner strength with every breath I take."

Sequence

1. **Mountain Pose (Tadasana)**
   - Stand tall with feet together, grounding evenly.
   - Center your breath and focus.
2. **Powerful Pose (Utkatasana)**
   - Inhale, bend your knees, and sweep arms overhead.

- Engage your core and sit deep into your strength.
3. **Forward Fold (Uttanasana)**
   - Exhale, hinge from the hips and fold forward.
   - Release the head and draw the nose toward the shins.
4. **Flat Back Lift (Ardha Uttanasana)**
   - Inhale, extend your spine, fingertips to shins or floor.
5. **Chaturanga Dandasana**
   - Exhale, step or jump back, lower down.
   - (Modify by lowering knees.)
6. **Upward Facing Dog (Urdhva Mukha Svanasana)**
   - Inhale, open the heart and lift the chest.
   - Thighs off the floor, shoulders back.
7. **Downward Facing Dog (Adho Mukha Svanasana)**
   - Exhale, lift the hips and press into your hands.
   - Find length in the spine.
8. **Warrior I (Virabhadrasana I)** – Right Side
   - Inhale, step the right foot forward, spin the back heel down.
   - Rise with arms overhead, hips aligned with back foot.
9. **Chaturanga Dandasana**
   - Exhale, lower down.
10. **Upward Facing Dog**
    - Inhale, lift heart, engage legs.
11. **Downward Facing Dog**
    - Exhale, send hips back.
12. **Warrior I – Left Side**
    - Inhale, step the left foot forward, back heel down.
    - Rise to Warrior I.
13. **Chaturanga Dandasana**
    - Exhale, move through the vinyasa again.
14. **Upward Facing Dog**
    - Inhale and standing on your hands.
15. **Downward Facing Dog**
    - Exhale and remain here for five full breaths.
16. **Flat Back Lift**
    - Inhale, step or jump forward to a flat back.
17. **Forward Fold**
    - Exhale, draw the nose to the shins.
18. **Powerful Pose**
    - Inhale, bend knees and rise back into Utkatasana.
19. **Mountain Pose**
    - Exhale, straighten the legs and return to center.

Benefits of Sun Salutation B

Physical

- Stretches and strengthens both the front and back chains of the body.
- Builds heat and cardiovascular endurance.

Energetic

- Stimulates prana (life-force energy) and enhances circulation.
- Balances solar energy through dynamic movement.

Daily Lesson Plan #12: Breathing Styles

Intention/Objective
Research various forms of breathing and their physiological effects.
Teaching Resource Materials
<ul><li>The Effects of Yoga on the Nervous System Handout</li><li>Namaskar Project Handouts</li></ul>
Review/Introduction
<ul><li>Discuss the Namaskar Project and set a date for submission in about two weeks so they have time to practice.</li><li>Distinguish between various forms of breathing, especially Yogic Breathing vs. Empowered Breathing and when and why we use each style.</li></ul>
Lesson
<ul><li>In groups of three, each group selects a sport or activity (from Pilates to singing) to research the type of breathing used and its specific purpose.</li><li>Students can then present their findings and have students practice the different types of breathing, followed by Q & A.</li><li>Discuss the two aspects of the Autonomic Nervous System- parasympathetic and sympathetic and how yoga influences the system.</li><li>Complete the class by having students lead three Surya Namaskar A's, the first one with their breath held as long as possible. Then do another while breathing through the mouth, with forceful exhalations. Finally, do a third Namaskar while breathing smoothly through the nose.</li></ul>
Reflection/Conclusion
Have you gained greater clarity on the importance of the breath and how subtle changes in breathing techniques influence the body/mind in very powerful ways?
OMwork
Observe your own breathing style and which aspect of your nervous system is activated most of the time. Place findings in your wellness portfolio.
OMwork Material
Four Types of Yoga Handout

The Effects of Yoga on the Nervous System

Adapted from the *Yoga for Diverse Learners Manual*

Yoga: More Than Physical Fitness

Yoga offers far more than increased strength, flexibility, and weight regulation. It has deep-reaching effects on our inner well-being, helping to:
- Calm a worried mind

- Focus scattered thoughts
- Promote emotional regulation
- Create a sense of inner peace and resilience

This profound calm is made possible through yoga's impact on one of the most vital systems in the body: *the nervous system.*

Understanding the Nervous System

The nervous system governs nearly every function in our body and mind. It can be divided into:

1. Central Nervous System (CNS):

- Comprised of the brain and spinal cord
- Acts as the body's main communication network
- Sends and receives messages to/from every part of the body

2. Peripheral Nervous System (PNS):

Divided into two major systems:
- **Sympathetic Nervous System (SNS)** – Activates during stress
- **Parasympathetic Nervous System (PNS)** – Activates during rest

The Stress Response: Fight, Flight, or Freeze

The **Sympathetic Nervous System** prepares the body to face perceived danger or challenge. It can be triggered by both real threats (e.g., a fire alarm) and daily stressors (e.g., crowded hallways).

Physiological effects of SNS activation:
- Increased heart rate and blood pressure
- Release of adrenaline and stress hormones
- Faster, shallower breathing
- Suppressed immune and growth hormone functions
- Increased oxygen demand and CO_2 expulsion
- Sweating and muscle tension

Note: Without time to rest and reset, chronic activation of this system can negatively impact physical and mental health.

The Relaxation Response: Rest and Digest

The **Parasympathetic Nervous System** supports recovery and calm. It becomes dominant during:
- **Yoga**
- **Conscious breathing**
- **Mindfulness**
- **Savasana** (relaxation time)
- **Social engagement**

Physiological effects of PNS activation:
- Lower heart rate and blood pressure

- Slower, deeper breathing
- Improved oxygen efficiency
- Strengthened immune function
- Relaxed muscles and mental clarity

> "I find it quite interesting that, with all the many wonderful and important things we learn in school, relaxation is stunted at our kindergarten graduation." — Nischala Joy Devi, *The Healing Path of Yoga*

Why This Matters

Yoga helps balance the nervous system by:
- Reducing stress hormones
- Boosting oxygen flow
- Enhancing mindful awareness
- Training the body to respond calmly instead of reacting impulsively

This is why quiet time at the end of class is essential. Savasana may feel unfamiliar at first, but over time, it becomes a welcomed time for peace and restoration.

Teaching Tip

Encourage students to build comfort with stillness and quiet reflection. Begin with a short Savasana (2–3 minutes), gradually increasing the time as students adapt.

The Four Types of Yoga

Yoga paths for different personalities and ways of learning.

Long ago, yogis realized that people connect with the world and grow in different ways. To honor this diversity, they developed **four main styles of yoga**, each suited to different personalities:

1. Jnana Yoga – The Yoga of Wisdom

"The Thinking Path"

Jnana Yoga focuses on **knowledge, self-inquiry, and inner wisdom**. Through questioning and reflection, Jnana yogis explore the difference between what is *real* and what is *illusion*. This is often considered the most intellectually demanding path.
- Goal: To discover one's **true self** by removing false beliefs and limiting patterns
- Practice: Study, contemplation, discussion, deep self-reflection
- Key teaching: *Discernment (viveka)* leads to liberation
- Example of a Jnana Yogi: **Swami Vivekananda**

Question:
Who else can you think of as a Jnana Yogi?

2. Bhakti Yoga – The Yoga of Devotion

"The Feeling Path"

Bhakti Yoga is all about **love, devotion, and surrender** to a higher power or purpose. This path channels emotion into spiritual growth.
- Practices: Chanting (kirtan), singing, **mantras** (repeating sacred sounds), prayer
- Goal: To open the heart and feel connected to something greater
- Common in yoga classes through **music and chanting**
- Example of a Bhakti Yogi: **Krishna Das (kirtan singer)**

Question:
Who else is a well-known Bhakti Yogi?

3. Karma Yoga – The Yoga of Action

"The Doing Path"

Karma Yoga is the path of **selfless service**. It teaches that every action can be a spiritual offering if done without expectation of reward.
- Practice: Helping others without needing credit
- Goal: Let go of ego by serving with love and purpose
- Example: **Mother Teresa** – a life of compassionate action
- Everyday example: Teachers, coaches, caregivers

"We must give our hands to serve, and our hearts to love." — Mother Teresa

Question:
Who in your life might be a Karma Yogi?

4. Raja Yoga – The Yoga of the Mind

"The Being Path"

Raja Yoga is the **"Royal Path"**, focusing on the mind-body connection and spiritual discipline. It includes **Ashtanga Yoga**, or the **Eight Limbs of Yoga**, which guide one to inner peace and unity.

The 8 Limbs of Raja Yoga

1. **Yamas** – how we treat others (non-violence, truthfulness, etc.)
2. **Niyamas** – how we treat ourselves (cleanliness, contentment, discipline)
3. **Asana** – physical postures (like in your yoga class!)
4. **Pranayama** – breath control
5. **Pratyahara** – turning inward, withdrawing from distractions
6. **Dharana** – focused concentration
7. **Dhyana** – meditation
8. **Samadhi** – blissful awareness, unity with all
- Practice: Regular yoga and mindfulness
- Goal: A quiet mind and a joyful heart
- Example: Patanjali – ancient sage who wrote the Yoga Sutras

Question:
Can you recognize how some of these limbs show up in your own yoga practice?

Daily Lesson Plan #12:
Breathing Styles

Reflection

Which style of Yoga do you relate to the most?
- **Thinking** (Jnana)
- **Feeling** (Bhakti)
- **Doing** (Karma)
- **Being** (Raja)

Yoga is not just about moving on the mat—it's a full-life practice that meets you wherever you are.

Namaskar Project

Curriculum Outcomes

By completing this project, you will demonstrate your understanding of the following:
- Perform Surya Namaskar A or B with proper alignment, integrating breath, asana, and movement.
- Apply effective breathing techniques to support your yoga practice.
- Show an understanding of anatomy and physiology in the intentional coordination of breath and movement.
- Identify yoga poses (asanas) for specific health benefits and use this knowledge to build a personal yoga sequence for use outside of class.

Project Instructions

You will work in groups of 3 or 4 to complete this creative assignment. Your task is to visually demonstrate your understanding of either Surya Namaskar A or Surya Namaskar B by creating a photo story sequence.

Steps to Complete

1. **Choose Your Sequence:**
   - Decide as a group whether you will represent Surya Namaskar A or Surya Namaskar B.
2. **Create a Photo Series:**
   - Each group member will be photographed demonstrating several poses in the sequence.
   - Ensure proper alignment and breath awareness is shown in the photos.
3. **Design a Poster (Bristol Board):**
   - Arrange the photos in the correct sequence of asanas.
   - Under each photo, include:
     - The name of the asana in both English and Sanskrit
     - Three ACE Alignment Tips (Alignment • Core • Extension)
4. **Examples of ACE Tips:**
   - **Alignment**: Stack shoulders over wrists in Plank Pose.
   - **Core**: Draw the navel to spine to activate Uddiyana Bandha.
   - **Extension**: Press through the heels to lengthen the back body.
5. **Presentation:**
   - Be prepared to share your project and discuss:

- How the breath supports movement.
- How your sequence benefits the body physically and emotionally.
- Any modifications used and why.

Alignment Rubric

ATTRIBUTE	0 POINTS STUDENT DISPLAYS:	1 POINT STUDENT DISPLAYS:	2 POINTS STUDENT DISPLAYS:	3 POINTS STUDENT DISPLAYS:
ALIGNMENT	No alignment	Insufficient alignment	Good alignment	Excellent alignment
ORDER/SEQUENCE	Incorrect order	Correct order		
LANGUAGE	Neither English NOR Sanskrit is provided	Either English OR Sanskrit is provided	Both English AND Sanskrit is provided	
CREATIVE VISUAL PRESENTATION	0 of the following: Neatness & clarity, effective class learning tool/display, colorful	1 of the following: Neatness & clarity, effective class learning tool/display, colorful	2 of the following: Neatness & clarity, effective class learning tool/display, colorful	3 of the following: Neatness & clarity, effective class learning tool/display, colorful
TEAM COLLABORATION	didn't work at all	worked independently	worked with some group members	included every group member

Namaskar Score

	Mountain	Powerful Pose	Forward Fold	Flat Back Lift	Chaturanga
Alignment					
Order					
English & Sanskrit					

	Upward Dog	Down Dog	Warrior 1-Right	Chaturanga	Upward Dog
Alignment					
Order					
English & Sanskrit					

	Down Dog	Warrior 1-Left	Chaturanga	Upward Dog	Down Dog for 5
Alignment					
Order					
English & Sanskrit					

	Flat Back Lift	Forward Fold	Powerful Asana	Extended Mtn	Mountain
Alignment					
Order					
English & Sanskrit					
TOTALS:					
OVERALL AESTHETICS MARK:					
				FINAL MARK:	

Daily Lesson Plan #13: Four Types of Yoga

Intention/Objective
Introduce four types of Yoga and inspire reflection on their preferred type of yoga.
Teaching Resource Material
Four Types of Yoga article, previously given as Omwork reading.
Review/Introduction
Ha=sun (action, warming part of poses), Tha=moon (easeful, cooling part of poses). Hatha Yoga describes the physical style of yoga that most of our western society is familiar with. It may come as a surprise to hear that Hatha Yoga is but one form that creates the grand discipline of yoga. Today we will explore the four main types of yoga.
Lesson
Discuss the four types of yoga. • Students can reflect throughout the class on which style of yoga particularly calls to their personality. **Centering:** • **Begin with a brief mindfulness practice.** Invite students to release any tension in and around the brain, allowing the mind to settle and quiet. Encourage them to gently begin breathing life into the body, from the inside out. • **Remind them that yoga is less about thinking and more about feeling**—a practice of becoming present and aware. Invite them to tune into the internal landscape of their bodies, noticing any areas of tension, discomfort, or ease. • This process of sensing the body from within is known as **embodiment**, or **interoception**—our capacity to perceive and respond to internal bodily sensations and needs. • **Encourage students to carry this awareness into their movement practice**, using it as a guide for how they move, breathe, and care for themselves on the mat. **Body of Class:** • Childs to Table to Thread the Needle, to gently stretch the neck and open the channels between mind and body. • Surya Namaskara A's (student led if anyone is ready) and • 3 Surya Namaskara B's, using Sanskrit terms where possible. • Introduce three variations of Standing Forward Folds that calm the nervous system: Padangusthasana, Uttanasana and Padahastasana. • Tree/Vrksasana • Staff/Dandasana to Seated Forward Fold/Paschimottanasana with a band around the balls of the feet if necessary. **Closing:** • Legs up the Wall/Viparita Karani, returning focus to softening the mind. Students may need to bend the knees or draw soles of the feet together etc. • Add soft music.
Reflection/Conclusion
What type of yoga are we doing when we practice asanas? Hatha Yoga, which is part of Raja Yoga. Chant Om Shanti, Shanti, Shanti, and Namaste your classmates.

Daily Lesson Plan #13:
Four Types of Yoga

OMwork
Journal entry to be assessed: Write a one-page, double spaced fictional story about one type of yoga, and include a teaching or moral message.
OMwork Material
• Affirmations for the Yamas • Article on the Path of Karma Yoga

Affirmations on Yamas

The following are affirmations that reflect the wisdom of the Yamas, moral guidelines:
   Ahimsa-kindness/non-harm: By challenging my limits, I learn where they lie and how to honor them. I am kind to my body, my bones, my muscles and my heart.
   Satya-truthfulness: I am honest with myself and that extends into my relationships. When I honor my truth, I live with integrity.
   Asteya- honesty/non-stealing: I don't take things that aren't mine. I let go of fear and scarcity. I breathe in love, honesty and trust.
   Brahmacharya-conservation of vital energy: I protect my energy by mindfully breathing and staying focused on the present moment, even through challenges.
   Aparigraha-generosity/non-hoarding: I move from greed and hoarding my possessions to an attitude of abundance. I loosen my grip and give and receive freely.

Karma Yoga – The Path of Selfless Service

Let's start with a simple question:
   What would truly bring us more happiness in life?
   At first, most of us might think of personal goals—like success, money, or comfort. Rarely do we say, "Helping others." But in the Yoga tradition, happiness isn't just about fulfilling our own desires. Instead, it asks us to reflect on two powerful questions:
   "Who can I serve?"
   "How can I serve?"
   These questions shift our attention away from ourselves and toward others—and that's the heart of Karma Yoga.

A Real-Life Reflection

Here's a story from one of my yoga students in training:

> "When I think about why I'm where I am in life, it comes down to service—what I do for others each day. I used to expect something in return for what I did, even if I didn't say it out loud. But now, I find so much joy in simply helping people. When someone smiles because of something I did, it fills me up. That's the best reward of all."

Many of us don't often act with **pure intention**—without hoping for a thank-you or something in return. But this student is describing the very essence of Karma Yoga:
giving without expectation.

Daily Lesson Plan #13:
Four Types of Yoga

Examples in the Community

Karma Yoga isn't just found in ancient texts—it's alive in our communities, too.
- A group of friends volunteers every Saturday at the soup kitchen on Gottingen Street. Over the years, they've built genuine friendships with the people they serve, helping create a sense of dignity and care in a space that might otherwise feel hopeless.
- Another example is a local fundraiser organizer who helped raise over $200,000 for a non-profit organization. He didn't do it for fame—just to make a difference.

These are everyday examples of Karma Yoga—**service from the heart**.

What Karma Yoga Teaches Us

Ancient yoga teachings say that when we give selflessly, life gives back—often in surprising ways. That same student later shared that after leaving a draining job to follow a more purposeful path, they began to feel truly fulfilled and at peace. Doors started to open, and life began to feel more meaningful.

Unfortunately, our culture often teaches the opposite:
"Find a good paying job."
"Get the job done, then live your life outside of work."
"Make sure every effort has a payoff."

This mindset can leave us feeling empty, fearful, or stuck. But when we shift to asking, "Who can I serve?" and connecting to the heart, we start to live with more **connection, joy, and meaning**.

Living the Karma Yoga Way

Yoga philosophy suggests we're each born with unique gifts—and we're meant to share them, not just use them for personal gain. This doesn't mean we need to give everything away or live without comfort. Many Karma Yogis live abundant, joyful lives because they've learned the natural rhythm of **giving and receiving.**

As the Dalai Lama said:

"Every day, think as you wake up: Today I am fortunate to have woken up. I am a precious human life. I am not going to waste it. I am going to use all my energies to develop myself and expand my heart out to others."

A Personal Invitation

Karma Yoga invites us to live with more **gratitude and generosity**.
Take a moment to imagine:
What would your life feel like if you gave freely—without needing anything in return?
Whether it's:
- Tutoring a younger student,
- Walking a neighbor's dog,
- Or simply offering a kind word—

Try an act of **selfless service** this week and notice how it makes *you* feel.
The joy of Karma Yoga is that by lifting others up, we rise too.

Daily Lesson Plan #14:
Yamas and Niyamas

Intention/Objective
To integrate the concepts of the Yamas and Niyamas into the students' practice and their lives.
Teaching Resource Material
Yamas and Niyamas Affirmations
Review/Introduction
<ul><li>Briefly discuss the Yamas and Niyamas as the first two limbs of Ashtanga Yoga (part of Raja Yoga), which are summarized in Sutra 11.30 and 11.32.</li><li>The Yamas support us with our interactions with others, focusing on our outer world, while the Niyamas support us with our inner world, helping us create a positive inner space from which to grow.</li><li>Understanding and applying these concepts are essential, for without this moral foundation, the practice of yoga is incomplete.</li></ul>
Lesson
Today the focus will be on kindness/Ahimsa, the leading and most important principle of the Yamas. Read Sutra 11.35. **Ahimsa Affirmation:** By challenging my limits, I learn where they lie and how to honor them. I am kind to my body, my bones, my muscles and my heart. **Centering:** Three silent Sun Salutation A's, noticing any forms that need modifications, in honor of Ahimsa. When they are done, students can reflect on their internal dialogue, the self-talk that consumed their Namaskara's. Without judgment, ask yourself if your thoughts are in keeping with Ahimsa and the affirmation. As a group, read the affirmation before proceeding through the remainder of the class. **Body of Class:**<ul><li>Powerful/Utkatasana to Forward Fold/Uttanasana flow, 3 times, like pushing off the top of a mountain on your skis. End the third cycle by hanging in Seaweed/Rag Doll and then into Padangusthasana with peace fingers hooked around big toes for five breaths.</li><li>Utthita Trikonasana/Extended Triangle, both sides, then return to Mountain Pose.</li><li>Partner Form: Practice against the wall, one at a time trying Triangle to Half Moon (Ardha Chandrasana) while the other adjusts the block beneath the grounded hand and encourages the opening in the hips.</li></ul>**Closing:**<ul><li>Pigeon/Eka Pada Raja Kapotasana with forehead resting on hands or a block.</li><li>Knees to Chest/Apanasana and squeeze every muscle as tight as you can and exhale release.</li><li>Savasana: Recite the Metta or Loving Kindness Practice:</li></ul>May I be healthy May I be happy May I feel safe May I dwell in peace.

• Rise to sitting and re-read the affirmation for Ahimsa: By challenging my limits, I learn where they lie and how to honor them. I am kind to my body, my bones, my muscles and my heart.
Reflection/ Conclusion
Observe your body's sensations and any uplifting side effects that your practice has had on your attitude.
OMwork
Practice Sun Salutation A and B first thing in the morning and record observations in your journal.
OMwork Material
• Sun Salutation B Script • Namaskar Project and Rubric Handouts

Giving New Light to a Dark Day

"By relating to others with respect and love (Ahimsa), we experience oneness."
– Yoga Sutra II.35

Even though many years have passed since the tragic events of September 11, 2001, (www.911memorial.org/learn/resources/911-primer/module-1-events-day) the date still carries a heavy emotional weight for many of us. This year, I woke up on the morning of 9/11 with a familiar feeling of sadness—but instead of sitting in grief, I asked myself:

How can I turn this day into something filled with peace and hope?

The answer came clearly and simply: **Project Hug.**

A Mission of Love

With my toddler, Sophia, in my arms, we set off to brighten our city—one hug at a time. Our first stop was the doctor's office. We chatted with people in the waiting room, but when it came time to offer a hug, I hesitated.

What if they think I'm weird?

I reminded myself of the purpose behind our mission: **to spread love.**

So, I approached the very professional-looking secretary and gently explained what we were doing. After a pause, she stood up, opened her arms, and gave me a warm, genuine hug. It was surprisingly meaningful—and something shifted inside both of us.

Next, we approached one of the doctors. He was reserved and formal, but after hearing our purpose and seeing Sophia on my hip, he also leaned in for a heartfelt group embrace. When we stepped away, we all had tears in our eyes. A shared moment of tenderness had taken root.

Feeling encouraged, we headed to Staples. After a kind young employee helped me find what I needed, I told him about Project Hug. He smiled, stepped in for a quick hug, and walked away with a bigger smile on his face than before.

Outside the store, I met a woman in a suit. "Because today is September 11th," I said, "we're offering free hugs." She lit up, gave me a tight squeeze, and said, "How nice!"

It really *was* nice—to connect, human to human, in our shared city.

At our final stop, the local market, I again heard that little voice:

Is this strange? Am I taking it too far?

But we pressed on.

We hugged a tall, joyful man in his 60s. We hugged a friendly woman who sells vitamins—someone who probably hugs people every day. We even hugged a woman in line who exclaimed, "I *love* this! I'm going to do it too!"

A Ripple of Positivity

By the end of the day, we had shared many small but powerful moments with strangers. Did we change the world? Maybe not. But maybe—just maybe—we helped soften the memory of a hard day. Maybe a few people walked away **feeling lighter**, **more seen, more loved**.

Your Turn: Practicing Ahimsa

You're invited to take part in your own version of **Project Hug**. The practice of *Ahimsa*—nonviolence, compassion, and love—asks us to step out of our comfort zones and connect with others in kind, respectful ways.

Always remember to be *trauma-sensitive* in your approach:
- Ask permission before offering a hug or physical gesture
- Respect all responses, whether yes or no

What's Your Plan?

What could *you* do to spread positivity today?
- A handwritten note?
- Helping a neighbor?
- Sharing your appreciation with someone who wouldn't expect it?

No act of kindness is too small. Like a hug on a hard day, it might just be the moment that turns someone's day—or even life—around.

Daily Lesson Plan #15: Peace Project

Intention/Objective
Collectively the class will identify a Peace Project and create an outline for the event.
Teaching Resource Material
Peace Project Handout
Review/Introduction
<ul><li>Review Ahimsa as the leading principle of the Yamas. How did the Metta practice go?</li><li>Have five students choose asanas from the posters as a warmup. The same five students can teach the asanas together, with the teachers' guidance if necessary.</li><li>Finish warmup with the Ahimsa Affirmation: By challenging my limits, I learn where they lie and how to honor them. I am kind to my body, my bones, my muscles and my heart.</li><li>Discuss the handout on Giving New Light to a Dark Day and how it applies to Ahimsa.</li></ul>
Lesson
Teachers can: <ul><li>Open the class for discussion about the Peace Project and offer a few suggestions for an event they will be organizing as part of the course.</li></ul> Some examples: <ul><li>Organize a Drumming and Yoga event with an Elementary School.</li><li>Organize a Community Yoga Fest for the community and host a guest teacher.</li><li>Climate Clean up - organize an environmental event where students promote the reduction of consumption, or the planting of a garden (or give a plant/tree to each student in the school), or drawing students awareness to their personal contribution to landfills by having a day where everyone carries their garbage in a bag around with them.</li><li>A day where students aim to break a record for the most random acts of kindness. They could visit a daycare, a children's hospital, or a seniors' home and present them with crafts that they've created or create them together.</li><li>School wide silent day with mindfulness practices at breaks and yoga at lunch, followed by a gathering at the end of the day with a guest speaker to close the event.</li><li>Agree upon a date for the event, identify tasks and timelines, arrange the roles of each student.</li><li>Make a list of things that would indicate a successful event (attendance, feedback, media exposure, interest in making it an annual event etc) and how the students will be assessed.</li><li>Select a few student leaders to supervise various tasks.</li></ul>
Reflection/Conclusion
Students can summarize details on chart paper with a "To do" list that can be checked off as tasks are completed.
OMwork
What needs to be done, by whom, and by when?
OMwork Material
Practicing Ahimsa Peace Project Handout Peace Project Rubric Peace Project Assessment

Proposal and Planning Process

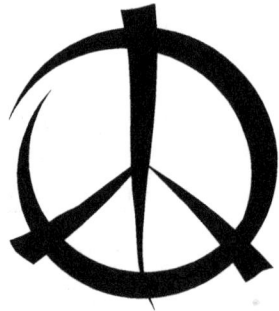

This project is aligned with the path of Karma Yoga, or Selfless Service.

Let's begin by asking ourselves what would bring us more happiness in life? Upon quick reflection, most of us would not respond with an answer such as helping others. The yoga tradition does not buy into the way of the ego that obsesses about every personal desire. When seeking more happiness and fulfillment, two of the highest questions we can ask ourselves are **"Who can I serve and how can I help them?"**

Brainstorm

Individually or with a partner, brainstorm to come up with three possible project ideas that will make a positive difference in your school or community. Once complete, get one of your ideas approved by your Yoga teacher.
1.
2.
3.

Get Approval

You must hand in a copy of your planning process, which includes the steps to organizing your project.
- Create a step-by-step document to identify the where, when, why and how this project will unfold.
- State the contact information to start your project. Include the name of the people you need to contact, the organizations, phone numbers and email addresses if available.
- When and where will your project unfold? How often will this event occur? How many hours are involved?
- What materials do you need, and how will you acquire them?
- What are the expenses and who will cover them?
- What is the meaning or intention behind your project?
- How will your project affect your participants?

Design a Form to Display the Following Information

Add any other categories that may seem appropriate for your specific situation.
- Name and location of organization of where you're conducting your Peace Project
- Indicate your audience/target group
- When & how many volunteer hours were completed

- Contact information for your supervisor (include phone number and email address)
- A section for your supervisor's comments after completing your service
- A signature from your supervisor

Sketch a Rough Draft of Your Form

Show what you will include in your form in the space below.

Your Reflection

This must be a minimum of two pages (double spaced). The purpose of this written work is to write a detailed essay of your overall experience. You should discuss the following:
- What was the main purpose of your project?
- If you worked with another person, document how the work was distributed.
- What was your favourite part of the project and why? How did you feel as a result?
- Were there any unforeseen challenges? If so, what would you do differently?
- Who should you thank and how can you express your appreciation?
- Who was impacted by this project? How and why?

Daily Lesson Plan #15:
Peace Project

Reflection Guidelines: Sharing Your Experience

Length Requirement: Minimum of two double-spaced pages.

The purpose of this written reflection is to thoughtfully explore your experience with your chosen project. Your essay should be personal, descriptive, and well-organized. Use the following guiding questions to help you build a detailed and meaningful response:

1. Purpose and Vision

- What inspired your project idea?
- What was the main purpose or goal behind your project?
- How did your project reflect your personal values or the values of the yoga philosophy (e.g., Ahimsa, Karma Yoga, community service, etc.)?

2. Collaboration and Teamwork (if applicable)

- Did you work with anyone else on this project?
- If so, how did you divide the responsibilities or tasks?
- How did the collaboration affect the outcome or experience of the project?

3. Personal Highlights and Emotions

- What was your favorite moment or part of the project?
- Why did this particular part stand out to you?
- How did it make you feel emotionally, mentally, or physically?
- Did the project change your perspective or inspire any new insights?

4. Challenges and Lessons Learned

- Were there any unexpected challenges or obstacles during your project?
- How did you respond to these challenges?
- If you were to do this project again, what would you do differently and why?

5. Gratitude and Acknowledgments

- Who supported you in completing your project (e.g., friends, family, strangers, teachers)?
- How can you show appreciation for their involvement or support?
- Why is it important to express gratitude in projects like this?

6. Community Impact

- Who was directly or indirectly impacted by your project?
- In what ways do you think it affected them?
- Do you think the positive impact will continue beyond the project? If so, how?

Final Note

Use clear paragraphs and examples throughout your reflection. Think of this as a story of your journey—include your thoughts, feelings, lessons, and the meaning behind your actions. Be honest, creative, and thoughtful. This is your opportunity to celebrate your work and the change it created, no matter how big or small.

Sample Reflection on Project Hug: Compassion into Action

The main purpose of my project was to bring light to a day that is often remembered with heaviness and grief—September 11th—by spreading love and positive energy through simple human connection. Inspired by the yogic principle of *Ahimsa*, or non-violence and compassion, I set out with my toddler to offer free hugs to strangers throughout our community. The goal was to transform a dark historical memory into a meaningful experience of hope, kindness, and unity.

Although I did not work with an official partner, I had a very important teammate with me—my young daughter, Sophia. Her presence helped soften every encounter and brought a sense of innocence and openness to the project that I could not have achieved alone. She was more than a passive participant; she was the heart of the experience. In many ways, people were more willing to engage because of her. While I initiated each interaction, Sophia was always by my side, reminding me of the purity and simplicity of love shared freely.

My favorite part of the project was seeing how open people became once they understood our intention. One moment that particularly stood out was hugging a reserved and professional doctor at our medical clinic. At first, he seemed closed off, but after hearing about Project Hug and seeing Sophia, he opened up—literally and emotionally. We shared a long, genuine embrace, and when we pulled away, there were tears in both our eyes. That moment reminded me of the deep human need for connection and how powerful small acts of kindness can be. I felt joy, gratitude, and a sense of purpose that stayed with me long after the hug ended.

Of course, not everything went smoothly. One of the unexpected challenges was my own hesitation. I found myself struggling with doubt and self-consciousness, worrying that people might judge me or feel uncomfortable. This fear nearly stopped me from fully committing to the project. If I were to do this again, I would take a moment before beginning to ground myself more deeply in the intention behind the project. I would remind myself that stepping outside of my comfort zone is a necessary part of growth—and that the discomfort is often temporary, but the impact can be lasting.

I would also like to extend heartfelt thanks to everyone who accepted a hug or smiled in response to our offer. I plan to send handwritten thank-you notes to some of the places we visited and will also share the story publicly in our local community forum as a way to celebrate the kindness we encountered.

The impact of this project was more widespread than I anticipated. While the individuals we hugged may not remember us forever, I believe the positive energy we shared rippled out through their interactions with others that day. A woman at the market even said she would start doing the same thing—imagine how many lives she may touch just by paying that intention forward. In a world that can often feel divided and isolating, these small moments of connection become incredibly meaningful.

In conclusion, Project Hug was more than a feel-good activity—it was a living practice of compassion, vulnerability, and service. It reminded me that changing the world doesn't always require grand gestures. Sometimes, a single hug or a moment of eye contact is enough to remind someone that they are seen, valued, and loved. This experience affirmed my belief in the importance of bringing yogic values into everyday life and inspired me to continue seeking ways to offer love freely and without expectation.

Peace Project Rubric

Points Awarded	1 point	2 points	3 points
How many ideas were established to offer peace?	1 idea	2 ideas	3 ideas
What level of detail was provided: where, when, why and how this project will unfold?	with minimal detail	with satisfactory detail	with great detail
Did the contact information include the following: supervisor's name, organization, phone number/ email address?	1 item included	2 items included	3 items included
Did the information form include the following: name, location, audience. Hours completed, supervisor's contact info, comments & signature?	Included some info	Included most info	Included all info
Does the student understand the meaning behind this project?	Understands some of the meaning	Understands most of the meaning	fully understands the meaning
According to the info provided, did the student contribute an equal portion to the group?	a partial contribution was made	an almost equal contribution was made	An equal contribution was made
Did the student provide an explanation of their overall experience including feelings & who was affected?	provided minimal explanation	provided a satisfactory explanation	provided an in-depth explanation
Was the student reflective and open to learning from the experience?	was minimally reflective and open	was somewhat reflective and open	was very reflective and open

Peace Project Assessment

Student Name:	
Requirement	**Score**
How many ideas were established to offer peace?	
What level of detail was provided: where, when, why and how this project will unfold?	
Did the contact information include the following: supervisor's name, organization, phone number/ email address?	

Daily Lesson Plan #15: Peace Project

Did the information form include the following: name, location, audience. Hours completed, supervisor's contact info, comments & signature?	
Does the student understand the meaning behind this project?	
According to the info provided, did the student contribute an equal portion to the group?	
Did the student provide an explanation of their overall experience including feelings & who was affected?	
Was the student reflective and open to learning from the experience?	
Comments	**Total**

Daily Lesson Plan #16:
Knowing & Speaking Your Truth/Satya

Intention/Objective
Students will consider the principle of truth and reflect on how it impacts their way of life.
Teaching Resource Material
<ul><li>Script for Classical Namaskar.</li><li>Small slips of paper for students to write on</li></ul>
Review/Introduction
<ul><li>**Affirmation for Satya-truthfulness:** I am honest with myself and that extends into my relationships. I honor my truth and live with integrity.</li><li>Check in by connecting to the breath and relaxing any tension spots. Notice any changes in your body or mind since the beginning of the course.</li><li>Discuss roadblocks like frustration or impatience etc. Today is an opportunity to be truly honest with yourself. How you do your yoga is how you do your life.</li><li>Ask yourself:<ul><li>Am I being honest about how much heart I'm putting into this course?</li><li>Am I being honest about the pain or discomfort I'm putting my body through?</li><li>Am I being honest about how present and mindful I'm being during practice?</li></ul></li><li>Through yoga we come to realize that the stories we've been telling ourselves about not being good enough, pretty enough, likable enough, are false. We come to realize that we are not broken, despite what others say about us.</li><li>As a group, the class can share (or not) some of the negative stories or lies they've been told about themselves that are not aligned with their deepest truth. These can be written on a sheet of paper and placed at the top of their mat. As the practice unfolds, students are encouraged to tear up their paper and toss it in the trash when they feel ready to release their false statement. Ideally all papers are gone by the time the class is over, but we can't force it.</li><li>Today, we are invited to let go of past hurts and false beliefs. We'll focus on tension spots and release held energy This class is designed to stretch the hamstrings through our Side Intense Stretch and Revolved Triangle.</li></ul>
Lesson
Centering:<ul><li>Breath awareness in Sukhasana.</li><li>Introduce Ujjayi Breathing with the slight constriction of the glottis, helping to slow the breath down and regulate our nervous system.</li><li>Seated Twist</li></ul>**Body of Class:**<ul><li>Introduce Classical Namaskaras and lead three on each side, six altogether. On the last ones, stay in the lunge for five breaths.</li><li>Powerful/Utkatasana to Standing Forward: Fold/Padangusthasana three times and linger in the final Standing Forward Fold for five or so breaths.</li><li>Mountain: Maintain awareness of your foundation in each standing asana, as this is your connection to the earth and to the truth.</li><li>Twisting Powerful/Utkatasana: Offer a rolled-up mat or prop for those whose heels lift. Hang in Rag Doll/Seaweed or Padangusthasana between the sides.</li></ul>

- With students in Mountain Pose (Tadasana), demonstrate the following sequence—or invite a student to model while you guide the class with verbal cues.
- **Transition from Mountain to Warrior I (Virabhadrasana I):** Step left foot back, bend the front knee and reach the arms overhead. Ground through the back heel and find length through the spine. What is your truth, are you living in a way that respects your needs, your truth? This requires the strength and courage of a warrior.
- **Move into Pyramid Pose (Parsvottanasana):** Straighten the front leg and bring the hands to the hips or behind the back. Begin to hinge forward from the hips over the extended front leg, keeping the spine long and both hips facing forward. Encourage students to stop where they feel a stretch without rounding the back too much.
- **Transition to Revolved Triangle (Parivrtta Trikonasana):** Place the opposite hand (from the front leg) on the floor, block, or shin outside the front foot. Extend the other arm toward the sky, stacking the shoulders. Encourage students to keep both legs strong and maintain a long spine. Offer the option to gaze up, forward, or down, depending on neck comfort.
- If time allows, repeat the above sequence and observe any differences the second time around.
- Standing Balance - Warrior 3/Virabhadrasana 3
- Downward Dog/Adho Mukha Svanasana to Child's/Balasana - knees together or apart, you choose. Begin to slow your breathing down, preparing to cool down.

Closing:
- Supine Twist/Jathara Parivartanasana variations for 10 breaths each side, letting go of held tension in the belly, neck or face.
- Savasana - repeat Satya/truth Affirmation: I am honest with myself and that extends into my relationships. I honor my truth and live with integrity.

Reflection/Conclusion

So many people speak untruths, especially today with political forums wrought with lies and false accusations of opposing parties. For many, lying becomes a habit. In yoga we are invited to speak our truth through Satya, while keeping Ahimsa/kindness top of mind. Just remember, what longs to be spoken finds its voice through practice.
Closing Quote: "Rather than love, than money, than fame, give me truth." Henry David Thoreau

OMwork

Epsom Salts baths relieve soreness in hamstrings and cleanse toxins.

OMwork Material

Read Article: Moment of Truth

Classical Namaskar/Salutation Script

Right Side

1. **Inhale** – Join hands together (Anjali Mudra)
2. **Exhale** – Bring hands to heart center
3. **Inhale** – Sweep arms forward and up (Extended Mountain)
4. **Exhale** – Hinge at the hips and fold forward (Standing Forward Fold)
5. **Inhale** – Step the **right foot** back into a lunge
6. **Retain the breath** – Step the **left foot** back into Plank
7. **Exhale** – Lower knees, chest, and chin to the mat (Coiled Serpent)
8. **Inhale** – Slide forward into Cobra
9. **Exhale** – Press back to Downward Facing Dog
10. **Inhale** – Step the **right foot** forward into a lunge
11. **Exhale** – Step the **left foot** forward; tuck nose to knees (Forward Fold)

12. **Inhale** – Rise with a flat back to Extended Mountain
13. **Exhale** – Sweep arms forward and down into Mountain (Tadasana)

Left Side

1. **Inhale** – Join hands together (Anjali Mudra)
2. **Exhale** – Bring hands to heart center
3. **Inhale** – Sweep arms forward and up (Extended Mountain)
4. **Exhale** – Hinge at the hips and fold forward (Standing Forward Fold)
5. **Inhale** – Step the **left foot** back into a lunge
6. **Retain the breath** – Step the **right foot** back into Plank Pose
7. **Exhale** – Lower knees, chest, and chin to the mat (Coiled Serpent or Child's)
8. **Inhale** – Slide forward into Cobra Pose
9. **Exhale** – Press back to Downward Facing Dog
10. **Inhale** – Step the **left foot** forward into a lunge
11. **Exhale** – Step the **right foot** forward; tuck nose to knees (Forward Fold)
12. **Inhale** – Rise with a flat back to Extended Mountain
13. **Exhale** – Sweep arms forward and down into Mountain (Tadasana)

Article: Moment of Truth

"The moment you accept what troubles you've been given; the door will open."
Rumi

Illusion and Awakening

Illusion refers to the deceptive world of the ego—a reality many of us inhabit unconsciously, day in and day out. It represents all that we are *not*, yet the egoic mind clings to this false identity for its survival. The ego thrives when we buy into the belief that we are separate from one another, and that our worth is determined by our appearance, career status, social circles, or material possessions. This illusion keeps us tethered to a life governed by surface-level values, rather than authentic truth.

Carl Jung once described personal growth as a transition from the "morning" of life, filled with ignorance and unconscious habits, to the "afternoon" of life, where we begin to awaken to wisdom and universal truths. In yogic philosophy, this shift is described as the journey from *avidya* (ignorance) to *vidya* (knowledge or wisdom). It is a sacred turning point—when we stop running from truth and instead face it with open eyes and a willing heart.

There comes a time in each of our lives when we are invited to meet truth face-to-face. And it is often through pain that this meeting occurs. When we find the courage to acknowledge the harder realities of our existence—without sugarcoating or denial—true healing and growth can finally begin.

For me, that moment arrived in the spring of my fourth and final year at Acadia. I had depleted every ounce of energy I had; my body was nearing complete collapse. One cold, misty Sunday, no longer able to run as I used to, I went for a walk. I wandered aimlessly through town and eventually found myself at the park. There, beneath the iconic weeping willow tree, I collapsed—exhausted, desperate, and alone. For the first time since developing anorexia, I offered an honest and wholehearted prayer for help.

In that moment, I surrendered. I admitted that my obsessive control, my tireless attempts to manage my brokenness, had not only failed to bring me peace—they had nearly cost me my life. For five long years, I had lived in the shadow of an illness that consumed my thoughts and distorted my sense of worth. As they say in Alcoholics Anonymous, I had been "boiled down to the bones"—stripped of all illusions and brought to the raw edge of truth.

Under the gentle drizzle of that rainy day, something within me shifted. For the first time in years, I experienced a desire to live. I lay on the grass and allowed myself to fully feel the truth of my pain—my loneliness, my shame, and my exhaustion. I cried—not because I was weak, but because I was finally strong enough to stop pretending. I realized that what I'd been seeking all along was not physical perfection, but love. I had made my relationship with food the most intimate one in my life, and it was not only unfulfilling—it was profoundly harmful.

In that moment of vulnerability, I acknowledged the roots of my suffering: the childhood trauma I hadn't dared to confront, the deep void left by emotional neglect, the pain of witnessing my parents' strained relationship, and the misplaced responsibility I carried for it all. I saw how my self-destructive habits were attempts to control or suppress what felt uncontrollable. But in allowing the truth to surface, I took the first step toward freedom.

That moment under the weeping willow marked the beginning of my healing. I chose to change teams—to take off the jersey of disease and stand with the part of me that wanted to live, to love, and to be whole. When we align with our highest self in this way, life begins to respond. New doors open. Unexpected grace appears. And from the depths of darkness, we begin to rise.

Daily Lesson Plan #17: Non-Stealing/Honesty/Asteya

Intention/Objective
Students will gain understanding of the principle of Non-Stealing/Honesty/Asteya.
Teaching Resource Material
Peace Invocation
Review/Introduction
<ul><li>Distribute or post hand out.</li><li>Honesty/Asteya Affirmation: I don't take things that aren't mine. I let go of fear and scarcity. I breathe in love, honesty and trust.</li></ul>
Lesson
Centering:<ul><li>Sit with your breath and this concept of non-stealing, even if you question or resist it.</li><li>Bee Breathing (Brahmari): Inhale through the nose and exhale with a humming sound, keeping mouth closed (similar to the sound of Om). Let the sound vibrate through your head, heart and body. This is likened to the sound that vibrates through the entire planet, through every being, every tree, every flower. Let it purify you, let it strengthen you, let it connect you to the abundance of life.</li><li>Based on our theme for today, create a personal intention or focus for your class, related to personal integrity and honesty.</li></ul>**Body of Class:**<ul><li>Classical Namaskar three times slowly.</li><li>Fourth Namaskar: Add tricep stretch to each lunge (right foot forward, left arm is up, hand behind head).</li><li>Fifth Namaskar: Add a basic twist to lunge (left hand to floor on inside of right foot, reach up with right arm).</li><li>Mountain, vinyasa to Downward Dog</li><li>High Lunge with arms overhead. Spend a few breaths here, with feet hip width for balance.</li><li>Lunge Twist, reaching left arm forward, right arm back for three breaths. Flow to the other side.</li><li>Revolved Side Angle: on the next lunge, lower back knee, and reach left elbow to the outside of the right thigh into Revolved Side Angle. Gradually lift the back knee if possible and bring hands into anjali mudra at the heart centre. Vinyasa to the other side.</li><li>Mountain to Powerful/Utkatasana to twisting Powerful/Utkatasana, by pressing the left elbow strongly into the right thigh.</li><li>Revolved side angle/Parivrtta Parsvakonasana: This time approached from twisting Powerful/Utkatasana by stepping left leg back into Revolved Side Angle.</li><li>Step forward and hang in a Rag Doll/Seaweed before entering the Standing Forward Fold/Padangusthasana.</li><li>Return to Mountain and switch sides.</li></ul>**Closing:**<ul><li>Seated Head to Knee/Janu Sirsasana to Seated Twist/Marichyasana C or Ardha Matsyendrasana on the same side, then switch sides.</li><li>Ananda Balasana or Half Ananda Balasana or a trauma-sensitive option, like supported Half Bridge/Setu Bandhasana</li><li>Relaxation/Savasana and read the Peace Invocation at the end of class.</li></ul>

Daily Lesson Plan #17:
Non-Stealing/Honesty/Asteya

Reflection/Conclusion
The practice of Asteya extends beyond just non-stealing material things, it includes stealing others self-respect, ideas (IP), homework etc. Can you think of other examples?
OMwork
Reflection: <ul><li>Take a moment to gently reflect on a time in your past when you may have taken something that didn't belong to you—whether it was an object, someone's time, ideas, or attention.</li><li>Acknowledge this without judgment. Offer yourself compassion, recognizing that at that point in your life, you may not have fully understood the impact of your actions. As Maya Angelou wisely said, *"When we know better, we do better."*</li></ul>**Writing Prompt:**<ul><li>Now, reimagine that same situation—but this time, let the story unfold from a place of greater awareness, guided by the principle of personal integrity and respect for others' belongings.</li><li>How do your actions change?</li><li>What impact does this have on you and those around you?</li><li>How does it feel to choose honesty and alignment with your values?</li><li>Let this story reflect who you are becoming and a step toward living more consciously in the world.</li><li>Add this to your wellness portfolio.</li></ul>
OMwork Material
Article on Asteya

Peace Invocation
Peace to this body,
Peace to this mind,
Peace to the rhythmic flow of breath,
Peace to the deep sea of feelings within.
May all beings dwell in safety and peace.
May there be a global culture of peace,
Communities rooted in peace,
And families guided by peace.
May our days unfold with peace,
Our nights rest in peace,
Our sleep be cradled by peace,
And our dreams be blessed with peace.
For the healing of every heart and soul,
May peace arise in each moment,
And be woven gently through all we do.

Article on Asteya-Non-Stealing/Honesty

Asteya Affirmation & Reflection Activity

You can print this out and place it beside each student's mat, display it on a Smartboard, or post it on the wall as a gentle reminder throughout the lesson.

Asteya Affirmation

"I don't reach for what is beyond my true needs. I release fear, inadequacy, scarcity, and control. I breathe in love, honesty, and trust."

Let's Reflect

What does it mean to say, "I don't reach for what is beyond my true needs"?
   This part of the affirmation encourages us to let go of the constant desire for more—especially when that desire is driven by comparison, insecurity, or greed. It can include things like spending more than we have, taking what doesn't belong to us, or grasping at attention or approval.
   Important note:
   This is **not** about settling for mediocrity or shrinking your dreams. It's about recognizing what is truly aligned with your values and purpose.

The Second Half of the Affirmation

Let's say it aloud together:
   "I release fear, inadequacy, scarcity, and control. I breathe in love, honesty, and trust."
   Each of the words we let go of—**fear, inadequacy, scarcity, and control**—feeds into a mindset of "not enough." This can lead to behaviors that reflect a stealing mentality: taking from others, dishonesty, or acting from desperation.
   When we feel safe, confident, and connected, we act with **integrity and generosity** instead.

From Guilt to Generosity

Stealing—whether it's a physical object, someone's idea, or their energy—often stems from feeling disconnected or "less than."
   It requires us to believe we are separate from others, which leads to guilt, shame, and a cycle of unworthiness.
   But through practicing **Asteya** (non-stealing), we move into a mindset of **abundance**:
- **Scarcity thinking:** "I'll never have enough, so I must take it."
- **Abundance thinking:** "I will work toward my goals with patience and trust. What I need will come."

Which path would you rather walk?
- **Stealing** = guilt, harm, and separation
- **Honesty** = empowerment, self-reliance and respect from others

When we begin to truly feel our interconnectedness with others, we understand that to harm or take from someone is to harm ourselves. In practicing **Asteya**, we choose respect—for others, for the world around us, and for ourselves.

Daily Lesson Plan #18:
Energy Management/Brahmacharya

Intention/Objective
Introduce Brahmacharya as a practice of honoring and conserving one's life force energy.
Review/Introduction
Management of energy/Brahmacharya Affirmation: I protect my energy by mindfully breathing and staying focused on the present moment, even through challenges.
Lesson
Centering: <ul><li>Lie on your back and **allow your body to soften**, surrendering into the support of the mat beneath you. Feel the grounding presence of the earth, and the quiet strength of the community around you. You are held. After a few centering breaths, place one hand on your lower belly and the other on your heart. Begin to attune to the subtle rhythm of your breath beneath your hands. Through yoga, we cultivate the art of listening—learning to connect to all aspects of ourselves, not by effort, but by presence. As you breathe, gently tune into the energy and wisdom held in these two powerful centres: your heart and your belly. Notice any sensations, emotions, or messages that arise. Simply witness—without needing to fix or change anything. Just listen.</li><li>This class will be focused on balance asanas to help sharpen our awareness of our breathing and the finer sensations, so we can see how we're using our energy.</li><li>Mountain</li><li>Sun Salutation A, three times</li><li>Sun Salutation B, three times</li><li>While in Downward Dog, notice where you are expending energy unnecessarily (like clenching the neck or breathing through the mouth). We can call these habits energy drains or thieves. Brahmacharya is about acknowledging that we only have so much energy and choosing to use it in ways that serve our wellbeing.</li></ul> **Body of Class:** <ul><li>Warrior 2/Virabhadrasana 2 to Exalted Warrior to Extended Side Angle/Parsvakonasana to Virabhadrasana 2 again, vinyasa to the other side, charging your system with each mindful breath. Standing Balance Asanas:</li><li>Warrior 3/Virabhadrasana 3</li><li>Dancer/Natarajasana</li><li>Side Plank/Vasisthasana, explain that the hands are called Hastas and the feet are called Padas in Sanskrit, and that this asasna balances on both the hastas and the padas.</li><li>Navasana in its three kramas/stages, from feet to the floor, to lifting feet with hands supporting legs to straight legs, arms parallel to the floor. Let this asana fuel your life force energy.</li></ul> **Closing:** <ul><li>Baddha Konasana/Bound Angle</li><li>Supta Baddha Konasana/Supine Bound Angle with the option to use a band around hips and feet.</li><li>Supported Half Bridge/Setu Bandhasana with a block under the hips and one between the knees.</li></ul> **Savasana:** <ul><li>**As you rest, notice the parts of your body that remain tense—even when there is no longer a need to hold on.** These unconscious patterns of contraction can linger out of</li></ul>

habit, often rooted in past stress or unprocessed emotion. Through the practice of conscious relaxation, you're learning to soften and dissolve holding patterns that quietly drain your energy. • In their place, you're creating space for healing energy to flow—nourishing your body, calming your mind, and restoring your sense of wholeness.
Reflection/Conclusion
Brahmacharya is the practice of energy conservation. To truly conserve our energy, we must cultivate love, respect, and appreciation for ourselves. These qualities form the foundation for setting healthy boundaries—with work, screens, toxic relationships, and other drains on our vitality. • This practice supports a life of longevity, clarity, and joy. • It's important to understand that Brahmacharya is not about being selfish. You can be both generous and discerning—offering your time and energy from a place of fullness, while also protecting your **prana** and your peace.
OMwork
• Identify the three main ways in which you drain your life force energy (screentime, poor nutrition, over-eating, sedentary lifestyle, partying etc). You may wish to re-read the assignment on Prana drains and gains. • Spend a day with one removed and record results. • Place findings in your Wellness Portfolio.
OMwork Material
Article on Brahmacharya

Understanding Brahmacharya: Energy, Moderation, and Respect

In the West, *Brahmacharya* is often narrowly interpreted as celibacy or sexual abstinence. While this is one possible lens, a broader and more practical understanding of Brahmacharya centers on **mindful use of energy**—practicing moderation in all areas of life, including but not limited to sexuality.

Another translation of this Yama is "to walk with the sacred." Traditionally, those who chose a monastic path were sent into solitude to dedicate themselves entirely to spiritual practice, channeling their energy inward and upward. It's worth noting that historically, these roles were reserved for men, while women were typically confined to domestic responsibilities. Thankfully, times have changed, and today all people can explore and embody spiritual practices in ways that honor their full humanity.

In a modern context, **Brahmacharya invites us to be intentional with our sacred energy**—to conserve it, direct it, and use it in ways that nourish our well-being and fuel our creativity. This approach is more realistic and affirming than the rigid suppression of desire that some religious systems demand. Suppressing natural human urges without understanding or support can lead to emotional imbalance and even harmful behaviors.

In ancient India, young people were advised to wait until they were mentally and physically ready before entering sexual relationships—something supported by modern neuroscience, which shows the brain continues developing into the early twenties.

Today, many young people are exposed to intense sexual messaging through media and peer influence, often before they have the tools or maturity to navigate these experiences in a healthy way. This can result in confusion, emotional distress, and boundaries being crossed.

In this class, you are encouraged to reflect deeply on your own sexual health. Consider your personal boundaries and how they support your **physical, emotional, and spiritual health**.

Brahmacharya isn't about shame—it's about **respecting yourself**, honoring your energy, and choosing moderation and mindfulness in a world that often pulls us toward extremes.

Daily Lesson Plan #19: Generosity/Aparigraha

Intention/Objective
Apply the principle of Aparigraha, or non-hoarding, to their personal practice and to life in a specific way of their choosing.
Review/Introduction
Activity: Exploring Aparigraha – The Art of Letting Go and Living Abundantly<ul><li>**Begin by giving each student a small, non-breakable item—like an eraser or pebble. Ask them to make a tight fist around it, palm facing down.**</li><li>**Now, ask them to slowly open their hand and let the item fall to the ground.**</li><li>"*Notice what happens when we grip tightly and then let go in this position—the object falls away. This represents a scarcity mindset—the belief that if we stop controlling or clinging, we'll lose everything.*"</li><li>**Next, have them pick up the item again, but this time, hold it in a relaxed hand with the palm facing upward. Ask them to gently open the fingers.**</li><li>"*What happens now? The object stays where it is. This symbolizes an abundant mindset— when we let go without fear, we can still hold what we value. There is trust, space, and ease.*"</li><li>**Now invite them to bring both hands together, palms cupped.**</li><li>"*Look at the shape your hands have made—a bowl, a vessel. Imagine how much you can hold when your hands are open, receptive, and generous.*"</li><li>**Reflection:**"*This is the heart of **Aparigraha**, or non-grasping. When we release the need to cling, hoard, or control, we make space to both give and receive. We begin to trust in the flow of life and tune into the truth of infinite abundance—in love, health, friendship, and even wealth.*"</li><li>"*As you hold this image of open hands, ask yourself: What am I ready to release? And what am I ready to receive?*"</li><li>**Generosity/Aparigraha Affirmation**: I move from greed and hoarding my possessions to an attitude of abundance. I loosen my grip and give and receive freely.</li></ul>
Lesson
Centering:<ul><li>Finger stretches: One at a time, starting with the pinky, then altogether, extension and flexion.</li><li>Stretch thumb to forearm.</li><li>Reach fingers wide, like spider hands and shake them out. "I loosen my grip and give and receive freely."</li></ul>**Body of Class:**<ul><li>Sun Salutation A two times, emphasizing the opening in Upward Facing Dog/Urdhva Mukha Svanasana.</li><li>Sun Salutation B with Dancing Warrior variation (lift leg up in Downward Dog, reaching right heel to left shoulder, and then step forward).</li><li>Next Sun Salutation B interlace fingers behind for Bowing Warrior to open the hips.</li><li>On the final Downward Dog, wave forward into Plank, and then into Wild Thing and make some NOISE.</li><li>Do this twice on each side, opening to the abundance of energy and enjoyment in the moment.</li></ul>

- Child's/Balasana and recite the affirmation.
- **Anatomy of backbending**: Explain that these asanas stretch the quadriceps and the psoas muscle in the hip, which are often associated with flexion, drawing inward for protection. Today we are opening the front body to explore new possibilities.
- **Table/Bharmanasana** to Balancing Table with right arm and left leg lifted, switch sides. Advance to taking hold of the left ankle with the right hand, arch and open. Switch sides.
- **Locust/Salabhasana** with arms alongside the torso, inhale and sweep arms and legs out like making a snow angel, exhale and tuck them in. Do this three times and squeeze and hold on the last one.
- **One Legged Frog/Bhekasana** (on belly, reach back and draw right heel to right outer buttock) to **Bow/Dhanurasana**
- **Camel/Ustrasana**, one arm at a time, then both arms reaching to catch heels (toes tucked).
- Recite affirmation, then sound out the exhalation and emphasize the concept of letting go.

Closing:
- Seated Head to Knee/Janu Sirsasana
- Seated Wide Legged Forward Fold/Upavistha Konasana with side stretch

Reflection/Conclusion

- When you loosen your grip, your trust expands and lets more light in.
- What are you setting free? (Scarcity thinking, self-doubt etc).

OMwork

Choose one of the asanas from this class and practice it each day up to 5 minutes. Journal about your experience.

Omwork Material

Aparigraha: The Art of Letting Go

Aparigraha: The Art of Letting Go

Aparigraha, the fifth Yama in the yogic tradition, is often translated as *non-possessiveness*, *non-grasping*, or *non-attachment*. Rooted in the Sanskrit word *"graha"* (to grasp), *"pari"* (on all sides), and *"a"* (non), Aparigraha encourages us to let go of the need to cling—whether to objects, people, ideas, or outcomes.

In a world that constantly urges us to acquire more—more things, more achievements, more likes—Aparigraha invites us to pause and ask: *What am I holding onto that is no longer serving me?*

Beyond Minimalism

While often associated with physical simplicity, Aparigraha goes deeper than decluttering your closet. It asks us to examine our internal attachments—expectations, fears, identities, and even emotional patterns. These "possessions" can weigh us down just as much as material ones.

Letting go doesn't mean we stop caring or striving. Instead, it's about creating space. When our hands (and hearts) are open, we are more able to receive what's truly meant for us.

How Aparigraha Shows Up in Daily Life

- **With Possessions:** Do I own this, or does it own me?
- **With Relationships:** Am I trying to control or manipulate others out of fear?
- **With Expectations:** Can I release the need for things to unfold a certain way?

- **With Self-Worth:** Am I defining myself by status, success, or appearance?

Living with Aparigraha doesn't mean becoming detached or indifferent—it means trusting that we are enough as we are, and that what is meant for us will come, and what no longer serves us can be lovingly released.

Practicing Aparigraha

1. **Gratitude Practice:** Gratitude naturally shifts our focus from what we lack to what we already have.
2. **Mindful Consumption:** Before buying or consuming, pause and ask: *Do I really need this? Why do I want it?*
3. **Digital Detachment:** Limit screen time, social media, or content that promotes comparison or craving.
4. **Journaling Prompt:** *What am I clinging to right now? What would it feel like to let it go?*
5. **Affirmation:** *"I release what no longer serves me. I trust in the flow of life."*

Living With Open Hands

When we embody Aparigraha, we begin to live with open hands—able to receive joy, love, and abundance without clinging. We loosen the grip of fear and scarcity and move toward freedom, peace, and deep inner trust.

Letting go, it turns out, isn't losing. It's making room.

Daily Lesson Plan #20: Review of Yamas

Intention/Objective
To summarize the Yamas.
Review/Introduction
Review the definition of each yama and speak out their affirmations together.
Lesson

Centering:
• Group Asana- Pinwheel
Yama Circle Game – Embodying the Ethics of Yoga
• **Set-up:**
   o Divide the class into teams of five.
   o Each team forms a circle, lying on their bellies with heads toward the center and enough space between each person.
   o Each student chooses one of the five Yamas to represent: **Ahimsa (non-violence), Satya (truthfulness), Asteya (non-stealing), Brahmacharya (energy conservation),** and **Aparigraha (non-possessiveness).**
• **How to Play:**
   o On your cue, the first student (representing the first Yama) stands up, clearly states their **Yama** and an **affirmation** that reflects its meaning (e.g., "I am kind in thought, word, and action" for Ahimsa), and walks *mindfully* around the circle, stepping gently between each person before returning to their spot.
   o Once they lie back down, the next Yama stands, shares their affirmation, and takes their turn walking the circle.
   o Continue until all five Yamas have been expressed, and the full circle is complete.
• **Optional Challenges:**
   o Add a playful competition element:
      ▪ Which team finishes first *in the correct order*?
      ▪ Which team best demonstrates the **spirit of the Yamas** through their movement, tone, and teamwork?
• **Debrief:**
   o After the game, gather the students to reflect:
   o What did you notice about the different Yamas?
   o Which ones feel easiest or hardest to embody?
   o How does it feel to physically move with intention and affirmation?
Body of Class:
• Sun Salutation A five times to symbolize the Yamas, reading the English/Sanskrit words and affirmation for each Yama at the beginning of the Sun Salutation.
• Have each student choose a Yama and then fill out a shape on their mat that reflects this principle (it doesn't have to be an asana).
• Divide the class into five groups. Give each group a Yama and take five minutes to create a group asana that depicts the meaning of the Yama (for example, Ahimsa might look like a group hug). Each group can present their asana to the class.
Closing:
• Silent Mindfulness practice: Breathing in for a count of four, breathing out to a count of eight for two minutes, returning to the breath repeatedly to calm the mind and the body.

Reflection/Conclusion
Trace one hand (hasta) on a sheet and label each digit with a Yama.

Daily Lesson Plan #20:
Review of Yamas

OMwork
<ul><li>Journal entry to be submitted and assessed: Reflect on the Yama that you would like to focus on for the next week. How will you make this principle a part of your daily life?</li><li>Design a creative art piece or find a song that reflects your Yama, as a reminder of this practice throughout the following week.</li></ul>
OMwork Material
Yama Creative Assignment

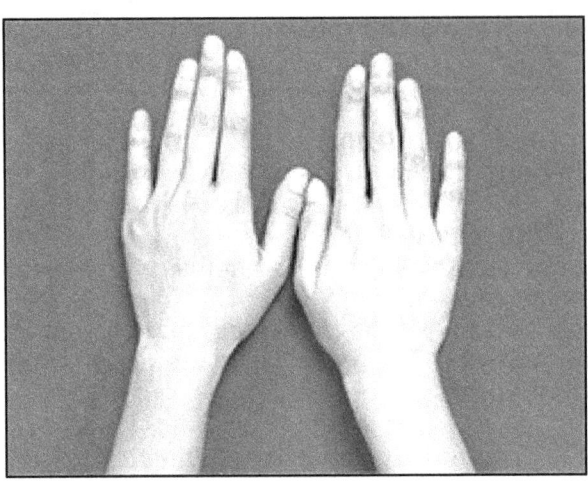

Yama Creative Assignment

Over the next week, choose **one Yama** (ethical principle from yoga philosophy) that resonates with you and commit to incorporating it into your daily life.

Reflection Journal Entry (Written Component)

Write a short journal entry that includes the following:
- **Which Yama did you choose and why?**
- Reflect on how this principle relates to your life right now. What draws you to it?
- **How will you live this Yama daily?**
- Be specific. Think about your routines, habits, relationships, and mindset.
- **How does your creative piece reflect this Yama?**
- Explain how your art will act as a visual or physical reminder to live by this principle.

Creative Component (Art Piece)

Design an original creative piece that represents your chosen Yama and will **serve as a daily reminder** of your intention.
   You may choose from the following ideas or get approval for something new:
- **Vision board** with images and quotes that embody your Yama
- **Locker poster** with visuals or affirmations
- **Collage** of personal or found images reflecting your Yama
- **Personalized place mat** to use during meals for mindful eating or gratitude
- **Bracelet or other jewelry** inscribed or designed with symbolic elements
- **Phone wallpaper** with an inspiring quote or image

- **Custom sticker for your water bottle** with your Yama's key message
- **Calendar reminder** (e.g., a daily alarm with a mantra, quote, or song that inspires your Yama practice)

Use this creative process as a chance to **connect deeply with your values** and create something meaningful that supports your personal growth.

At the end of the week, be ready to share how the practice influenced your mindset or actions.

Yama Rubric

Requirement	Points
Artwork does not display effort, reflection & creativity to represent chosen Yama	0-2 Points
Artwork displays insufficient effort, reflection & creativity to represent chosen Yama	3-4 Points
Artwork displays satisfactory effort, reflection & creativity to represent chosen Yama	5-6 Points
Artwork displays very good effort, reflection & creativity to represent chosen Yama	7-8 Points
Artwork displays excellent effort, reflection & creativity to represent chosen Yama	9-10 Points

Student Name:	
Chosen Yama	**Score**

Daily Lesson Plan #21: Introduction to Niyamas and Purity/Saucha

Intention/Objective
Students will gain understanding of the concept of purity of body, mind and emotions.
Teaching Resource Material
Handout article on Transforming Toxic Relationships with Saucha.
Review/Introduction
Niyamas are personal practices that strengthen our character and support our wellbeing. **Saucha Affirmation:** I choose my thoughts, words and actions carefully, so that my behavior helps me, and others to feel good.
Lesson
Centering: • Discuss Saucha as a cleansing practice, not just physically but mentally and socially as well. Chat about how easy it is to join in on hurtful gossip, poor lifestyle habits or destructive thinking about oneself when in the presence of peers. These habits all create toxins (stress hormones) in our systems. • **Saucha: Mental Practice - Pratipaksha Bhavana/transforming thoughts:** Think of a recurring negative thought that leads you to feel badly about yourself. Now question its truth by imagining that the opposite was true. Create an opposing statement or affirmation that can replace this negative thought when it appears in the future. For example: a negative thought "I have such huge thighs, they're disgusting!" to a positive affirmation "My thighs are amazingly strong, and I choose clothing that compliments my curves." • **Saucha: Social Practice:** Reflect on a social scenario in the past that has been hurtful or painful to a peer. Create an action step for practicing Saucha in social situations that would inspire better feelings. For example, instead of poking fun at a weaker player on your team, you could choose to be silent and not engage or even step in to support. **Body of Class:** • **Saucha: Physical Practice – Nauli:** It is known in yoga that what we consume becomes our physical state. This exercise helps to stimulate our systems of digestion and elimination. • In Mountain, inhale arms overhead and exhale hinge at the hips. Bend the knees and place hands on the thighs. Keep exhaling until the lungs are empty, then lift the abdominal organs up under the ribcage like a vacuum. Hold the exhalation as long as possible and then release the belly and inhale. Take a few breaths and try again. This exercise massages the internal organs and stimulates their natural functions. • Move through five to ten silent Classical Namaskar, using the rhythm of your breath to purify your body and mind. • Yogic Squat/Malasana for five breaths, three times. **Closing:** • Pigeon/Eka Pada Raja Kapotasana: Make this asana as challenging as you wish by sliding the tucked foot up toward the front of your mat. Let the exhalation carry away any stuckness in the tissues of the hips. • Savasana - take this time to release negativity in your thoughts and words and let go of destructive habits. When we feel good about ourselves, we become more attractive and our positive energy uplifts everyone around us.
Reflection/Conclusion
Saucha helps us to cleanse our systems so we can experience what it's like to live as a yogi: Light, graceful, serene, joyful and healthy.

Daily Lesson Plan #21:
Introduction to Niyamas and Purity/Saucha

OMwork
Apply your affirmation to your life and journal about its effectiveness. And remember, the process of changing habits takes determination and patience.
OMwork Material
Read article on Transforming Toxic Relationships with Saucha Affirmations for Niyamas

The following are affirmations that reflect the wisdom of the Niyamas, or positive habits:

- **Saucha-purity:** I choose my thoughts, words and actions carefully, so that my behavior helps me and others to feel good.
- **Santosha-contentment**: Breathing in, I am content with this moment. Breathing out, I am at peace with myself.
- **Tapas-self-disciplined effort:** Through daily practice and self-discipline, I enjoy radiant health and the fulfillment of my dreams.
- **Swadhyaya-self-inquiry:** When I pay attention to myself, the right answer emerges within me.
- **Ishvara Pranidhana-trusting the process:** I surrender to the Love Intelligence that is around me and within me, supporting me always.

Together the Yamas and Niyamas remind us to live with decency and respect, as we make choices that enhance the welfare of all beings.

Transforming Toxic Relationships with Saucha, Q & A with Jenny and Blair

Question

What do you do when friends gossip about others, but then act nice to those same people's faces? I try not to join in, but it feels awkward. It also makes me wonder—would those same friends talk behind my back too?

Blair

Unfortunately, this kind of situation is all too common, especially at school. It reminds me of a quote from the Dalai Lama: "If you can, help others. If you cannot do that, at least do no harm." Imagine how different the world would be if we all followed that simple rule.

Since that's rarely the case, my first piece of advice is to step away when the negativity starts. You don't have to stay in conversations that bring you down—even if you're not participating, the bad energy can still affect you. Trying to change the subject constantly can also backfire, creating tension or making you the next target of complaints, so be careful with that approach.

I've faced similar challenges and found it helpful to focus on positive activities instead. For example, I'd use my lunch break to get fresh air by walking around the neighborhood, soaking in the good vibes from the community.

But don't isolate yourself completely, maintaining some connection is important. You can influence your environment by disengaging from the negativity and modeling respectful, positive interactions.

Jenny

Toxic relationships really do affect our well-being. Time is precious, and it's great that you're considering how you're spending it.

When people have different perspectives, it's helpful to approach the situation with compassion. Gossip often comes from a place of insecurity, some people would rather bond over negativity than feel lonely.

I've been in groups where the conversation suddenly turns harsh and critical about someone else. Toxic talk can escalate quickly, so it's important to be clear about the kind of conversations you're willing to engage in. Also, spreading harmful comments only causes more pain, so practicing mindful communication benefits everyone.

By sticking to your intention to build healthy connections, you'll likely find people drawn to you because you offer a safe and respectful space. Eleanor Roosevelt said, "Great minds discuss ideas. Average minds discuss events. Small minds discuss people." Be that great mind!

As for worrying about people talking behind your back, remember the saying: "What other people think of you is none of your business." You can't control what others say or think, but you can control how much you let it affect you.

Let yoga fortify your strong foundation of self-worth and confidence, so other people's opinions just slide off you like water off a duck's back. Before entering difficult conversations, take a deep breath and remind yourself that you are a person of integrity, living in alignment with your highest values.

Saucha Affirmation:

I choose my thoughts, words, and actions mindfully, so that my behavior uplifts myself and others.

Daily Lesson Plan #22: Contentment/Santosha

Intention/Objective
Students will gain awareness of what contentment and lack of contentment feels like, with a movement practice focused on Contentment/Santosha.
Teaching Resource Material
Handout the article on The Grip.
Review/Introduction
<ul><li>**Santosha Affirmation**: Breathing in, I am content with this moment. Breathing out, I am at peace with myself.</li><li>Discuss the feeling of not being content (striving, competition, comparisons, need to please, doing, living in the past or the future etc). As the old saying goes, suffering comes from wishing we were somewhere, or someone else.</li><li>There is a term called 'The Grip' that describes this state of discontentment within the body. See hand out.</li><li>One way to describe contentment is the art of living in the present, which is the foundation of a mindful practice.</li><li>What other terms could be used to describe contentment? (satisfaction, peace, being etc).</li></ul>
Lesson
Centering:<ul><li>Practice stop and wait breathing by finding stillness, focusing on the breath and seeing what happens. This simple process helps to identify your specific areas of tension and allow the energy of contentment to soak into your body.</li></ul>**Body of Class:**<ul><li>Seated Jelly Fish with hands on knees, add a hug as the spine curls in.</li><li>Windshield wipers: sitting with hands behind, feet on floor in front with knees bent, sweep knees from side to side.</li><li>Table/Bharmanasana with Cat/Cow undulations.</li><li>Downward Dog/Adho Mukha Svanasana, to Plankasana three times.</li><li>Plankasana to Side Plank/Vasisthasana with upper arm circles, both sides.</li><li>Child's/Balasana, release the grip and breathe.</li><li>Standing Breath of Joy for five to ten cycles, letting yourself be enough.</li><li>Standing Forward Fold/Padangusthasana with full acceptance of your body</li><li>Warrior 2/Virabhadrasana 2 to Extended Triangle/Trikonasana to Standing Half Moon/Ardha Chandrasana, back to Triangle/Trikonasana.</li><li>Standing Wide Angle Forward Fold/Prasarita Padottanasana</li><li>Standing Balance Asana: Extended Hand to Toe/Utthita Hasta Padangusthasana (modified or full version).</li><li>Encourage students to practice their Drishti to focus their wandering minds, by softly gazing at a spot in front that's not moving.</li><li>Staff/Dandasana, practicing acceptance of self.</li><li>Partner Asana: Seated Forward Fold/Paschimottanasana</li></ul>**Closing:**<ul><li>Restorative asana of students' choice, such as Supine Twist or Knees to Chest.</li></ul>

Daily Lesson Plan #22: Contentment/Santosha

Reflection/Conclusion
Reflect on how much of your life you spend wishing you were somebody else, or somewhere else. Applying the practice of Santosha brings more peace into our lives, as we practice being content with this imperfect, beautiful life that we are privileged to live.
OMwork
Explore the areas in which your body holds tension. If 'The Grip' could talk, what would it say to you?
OMwork Material
The Grip article

The Grip

Have you ever taken a moment to notice how your body is holding itself right now? In yoga and mindfulness practices, we learn to relax the body by tuning into the breath and guiding its natural flow. The goal of Yoga—especially pranayama, the art of breath control—is to create a smooth, steady rhythm that calms the mind and releases deep-seated tension.

Yet, there's something that can slow down this process of calming the mind, often called 'The Grip.' This refers to areas of physical tension that tend to settle in one or two spots in the body. Everyone's Grip is unique—its location and strength shaped by our life stories, relationships, stress, and past traumas.

The Grip represents our fear-driven, protective thoughts made manifest in the body. These thoughts, often linked to the ego, convince us that we are separate from others and push us to judge or criticize, widening that sense of separation. The Grip not only tries to shield us from the perceived dangers of the outside world but also keeps the outside world at bay from the 'threats' it believes are inside us. The Grip may also be an appropriate response to a direct attack on one's safety, so it may have served you well at a point in your life.

Each of us carries tension differently—some hold it in the belly, others in the neck, and many feel it in the head. Wherever your Grip lies, it likely formed for a reason. For example, one yoga student who faced verbal abuse as a child—being told she would never succeed because she was female—holds tension in her lower abdomen, near her womb. Another, who suffered a concussion as a child while playing hockey, carries persistent tension behind his eyes.

The Grip is a clever defense mechanism, but it has a downside. Tension and pain cause blockages in energy flow and circulation. Where energy can't move, life force diminishes. Releasing your Grip allows energy to flow freely again, bringing life back to those tight areas. As your body softens, what you've been holding onto begins to let go and freedom fills the space.

When the body unwinds and energy channels reopen, fatigue and illness lessen, and vitality returns. It's that simple—and that profound. This is the true transformative power of yoga.

Daily Lesson Plan #23:
Balancing Effort/Sthira and Ease/Sukha

Intention/Objective
To apply the balancing principles of effort and ease to asana practice.
Teaching Resource Material
Image of an old fashion scale or a teeter totter.
Review/Introduction
<ul><li>Many people live with excessive stress and overexertion, whereas others are under stimulated and sedentary. In the Yoga Sutras there are two terms that describe the balance of these two dynamic energies. In Sutras 11.45 and 11.46, Patanjali refers to Sthira and Sukha, or steadiness and ease.</li><li>Sthira/steadiness is the effort that builds strength and Sukha/ease is the relaxation that restores our energy.</li><li>When we heavily emphasize effort, we try too hard in our yoga practice, which leads to fatigue and possible injury.</li><li>When we're lazy in our asanas and don't put forth enough effort, we miss out on the benefits of the practice, such as muscle strength and cleansing.</li><li>This concept is often referred to as two wings of a bird which cannot fly smoothly if there is imbalance.</li><li>In our practice today, we will be seeking opportunities to explore the balance of effort and ease in each asana. The goal is to find effortless effort, which is found when we discover true alignment in the asana, where the proper muscles are engaged while the others are at ease and lengthening.</li><li>Sthira and Sukha Affirmation: "I balance my effort with ease in every movement."</li></ul>
Lesson
Centering: <ul><li>Take a moment to consider that your heart is in a constant dance between Sthira and Sukha, contracting as it beats, relaxing in the pause. The same rhythm is found in our breath flowing in and out, and in the day versus the night.</li><li>In partners, do five Sun Salutation A's with just breath guidance or in silence, reciting quietly the affirmation 'I balance my effort with ease in every movement'.</li><li>Discuss anything that you observed as different.</li><li>Do five Sun Salutation B's as a class and discuss.</li><li>Where do you tend to over-exert?</li><li>How are the asanas different when you soften and let it flow?</li><li>Where do you not engage properly or wander mentally?</li><li>How are the asanas different when you focus on effective muscular engagement?</li></ul> **Body of Class:** <ul><li>Tree/Vrksasana</li><li>Standing Half Lotus/Ardha Baddha Padmottanasana</li><li>Yogic Squat/Malasana</li><li>The Crow/Bakasana with blocks in front for support, balancing effort and ease.</li><li>In partners, choose one or two asanas that you each find challenging. Lead yourselves into and out of these two asanas and seek to find the balance of effort and ease.</li></ul>

Daily Lesson Plan #23:
Balancing Effort/Sthira and Ease/Sukha

Closing: • Savasana: Progressive relaxation, squeezing your muscles tightly and over-emphasizing effort, allows you to deepen your experience of ease. • Savasana is all about EASE and releasing remaining muscular effort.
Reflection/Conclusion
Sitting mindfulness for 1-2 minutes, reciting the affirmation. Visualize yourself re-entering your life with the balance of effort and ease.
OMwork
Read Sutras 11. 45 and 11.46 and explore the duality of effort and ease on and off the mat. What needs to be revised in your life to find better balance? What do you notice about our culture with regards to effort and ease? Report your experience in your wellness portfolio.

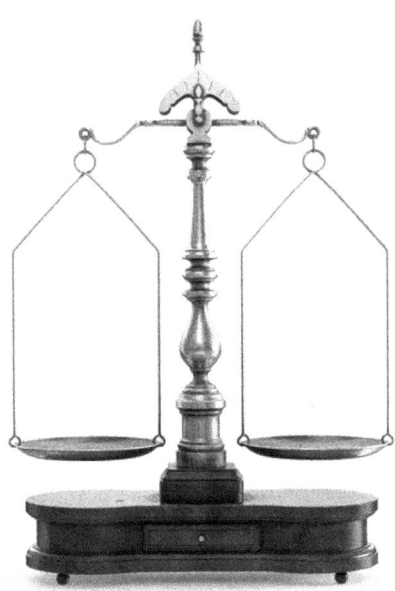

Daily Lesson Plan #24: Igniting Heat/Tapas

Intention/Objective
To ignite the heat of tapas and recognize its value in practice.
Teaching Resource Material
Tealights for each student. **Note of caution:** Battery operated candles can be injurious when they are stepped on so proceed around the room with caution.
Review/Introduction
<ul><li>**Tapas affirmation**: Through daily practice and self-discipline, I enjoy radiant health and the fulfillment of my dreams.</li><li>Through the practice of mindfulness and asanas, we develop Tapas, also described as 'heat', which brings transformation through discipline. Tapas is also cultivated through lifestyle choices: how we eat, sleep and socialize. Self-discipline is a significant part of our practice together, as the eventual goal is to sustain a personal daily practice on your own.</li><li>Just to be clear, Saucha is the practice of cleanliness and purity, while tapas is the practice of self-discipline or burning enthusiasm.</li><li>Self-discipline is a virtue that not everyone naturally has, and therefore, it must be taught and encouraged, especially with so many industries preying on our attention.</li><li>Self-discipline is required to pursue our dreams and experience personal satisfaction.</li><li>Who are a few people you see practicing self-discipline within their lives? (athletes, scholars, musicians, entrepreneurs etc).</li><li>What are they able to accomplish with their passion?</li><li>What sacrifices do you think they have to make?</li></ul>
Lesson
Centering:<ul><li>Introduce the class to Kapalabhati. Lead two sets of thirty breaths with easy breathing between rounds. One hand on the belly may help them force the air out like a bellows.</li></ul>**Body of Class:**<ul><li>Classical Namaskaras six times with a constant flow, no rests in Downward Dog or in Mountain.</li><li>Mountain/Tadasana for five to ten breaths, notice how you feel and observe the heat/Tapas in your body. Acknowledge the self-discipline that was needed to override any doubting inner voices to complete these Namaskaras. You just practiced Tapas!</li><li>**Core work**: Plankasana on elbows, inhale and lift core, exhale reach out from crown to heels for 1 minute. Do these two to three times.</li><li>Low lunge with Tricep stretch/Anjaneyasana. Transition to the other side with "Lion Climbing Mountain", by scissoring the legs six times, lifting the hips high through the transition.</li><li>Puppy Asana for five breaths, (Child's with the hips over the knees and arms outstretched in front). Let the head hang and rest on the floor if it will.</li><li>Dolphin/Pincha Mayurasana Prep, leaning the torso forward and back for ten cycles.</li><li>Side plank/Vasisthasana to Wild Thing/Camatkarasana for five breaths. Build the heat in the core with each breath.</li><li>Half Bridge/Setu Bandhasana with arms sweeping overhead as hips lift and lower, three to five times.</li><li>The Bow/Dhanurasana or repeat Half Bridge/Setu Bandhasana.</li><li>Partner Falcon: partner A lies on their back and balances partner B in the air by placing feet at their hip creases and holding their hands. Visualize yourself flying to new heights and achieving your goals with the determination and discipline of Tapas.</li></ul>

Closing:
• Knees to Chest/Apanasana or Ananda Balasana for five to ten breaths
• Relaxation/Savasana
Reflection/Conclusion
Tapas awakens our core and ignites our metabolism, making all of our body's systems more efficient, including the assimilation of food and elimination of waste.
OMwork
• Journal about something you've always wanted to achieve but didn't have the discipline or belief that you could do it.
• Write it down, read it daily and share it with a trusted source.
• For the next class, bring in an item that inspires peace and comfort.
OMwork Material
• Article on stoking your inner flame and cultivating Tapas
• Article on Practice and Tapas/self-discipline

Igniting Your Inner Flame: Cultivating Tapas

One of my fondest childhood memories of winter is stepping into my grandfather's century-old house after hours spent playing outside. As the door creaked open, a comforting wave of warmth from the wood stove mixed with the inviting scent of freshly baked ginger cookies would greet me. That wood stove, standing at the heart of his home, was the center of winter life—where meals were cooked, mittens dried, and hearts warmed as we gathered around, sipping hot chocolate in rocking chairs. According to Ayurveda, an ancient healing system, our wellbeing depends on keeping our internal stove burning brightly, especially through the cold months.

Winter can be challenging for all living beings in cold climates. Animals prepare months in advance—storing food, adding body fat, and building snug shelters. Humans have their own rituals, mostly focused on protecting our belongings: covering outdoor furniture, changing tires, and stocking salt. But surviving winter also means caring for our physical health. Viruses thrive in stagnant air, and our immunity weakens in cold weather.

One of the best ways to guard against winter illnesses is to keep your body warm and metabolism strong. Here are five yogic tips to help stoke your inner fire:

1. **Protect Your Extremities:** While most of us bundle up during the cold months, don't forget that heat escapes easily through your hands and head. Always wear gloves and a warm hat that fully covers your head—sorry, baseball caps don't count!
2. **Warm Liquids:** A teacher of mine always carries a thermos of herbal tea. Sipping warm liquids like ginger or chai tea throughout the day keeps you hydrated and supports your immune system far better than that rushed morning coffee.
3. **Digestive Elixir:** Boost sluggish digestion with a homemade digestive tonic. Try mixing ½ cup ginger juice, 1 cup lemon juice, ½ cup water, ¾ cup honey, ¼ teaspoon black pepper, and a pinch of cayenne pepper. Blend and enjoy throughout the week!
4. **Daily Movement:** Exercise is the ultimate way to spark your metabolism and generate lasting internal warmth—far beyond what any winter coat can offer. Sweating after a workout also helps detoxify the body (this is tapas in action). Starting your day with movement keeps your inner fire burning all day long.
5. **Mind Your Posture:** Notice how your body tenses up when rushing through the cold—head forward, shoulders rounded, stiff and tight. When your internal fire burns steadily, you'll naturally stand taller, breathe more freely, and feel relaxed and balanced.

By following these simple steps to keep your inner flame alive, you can enjoy the vitality and joy of life even in the coldest winter days.

Practice and Tapas (Self-Discipline)

As you progress through this program, it's normal to sometimes feel bored with the repetition of routines and exercises. We live in a world that constantly pushes us to seek new and exciting experiences. But pause for a moment and consider what top athletes, actors, surgeons, or master chefs all share: they've all dedicated countless hours to practicing their craft, refining their skills repeatedly. To reach mastery or achieve vibrant health, we must be willing to do what many won't—commit to consistent practice, even when we feel discouraged or frustrated.

This steady commitment is what yogis call *tapas*—self-discipline that's detached from the outcome. The beauty of yoga practice is that no matter your individual goals, it supports your deepest desires through focused attention, discipline, and purposeful effort.

Practice by nature involves repetition and dedication. It's like digging a deep well instead of a shallow pool. You repeat the fundamental skills until they become second nature, then build on them step by step. Eventually, you may find that poses like Downward Dog become a place of ease, your movements flow with unexpected grace, your arm balances feel stable, or your reactions to challenges become calmer.

The secret to growth lies in approaching mindful practice with a fresh, beginner's mind each day. For someone new to yoga, daily practice might feel repetitive or dull. But the mindful practitioner understands that every day is different—the body ages, the seasons change, the moon shifts, and the sunlight falls differently. Every moment is unique, sacred, and impossible to repeat. By embracing this, you develop tools that enrich your life deeply.

Starting a practice can be challenging—finding the time, setting your alarm, overcoming excuses. But once you create a routine—knowing that between 2:00 and 3:00 pm you have yoga with familiar people, the same teacher, and your own mat—you establish a rhythm. Over time, this practice becomes a nourishing part of your day, something you anticipate and protect.

This is the paradox and the gift of practice: doing the same thing repeatedly, but with curiosity and openness, recognizing that the benefits—physical, mental, and spiritual—may take time to appear but they're worth it.

Reflecting on your yoga journey so far, what insights have you gained about *tapas*, self-discipline, practice, and growth?

Daily Lesson Plan #25:
Self-reflection/Swadhyaya

Intention/Objective
To affirm the importance and benefits of personal growth and study of the self.
Review/Introduction
<ul><li>Students will have brought in an inspiring item from home and journals.</li><li>**Self-reflection/Swadhyaya Affirmation**: When I pay attention to myself, the right answer emerges within me.</li></ul>
Lesson

Centering:
- Sit comfortably and take a moment to repeat the affirmation that reflects the practice of self-study/Swadhyaya - When I pay attention to myself, the right answer emerges within me.
- Swadhyaya helps us to better understand ourselves; the way our body works, our emotional triggers and moods, as well as our reactions to various life situations and people. Through our practice of self-inquiry, our awareness moves from knowledge to knowingness.
- Mountain
- Sun Breaths, three to five times.
- The Phoenix: step left foot behind the right and reach left elbow across chest. Extend your right arm up and gaze up, rooted and yet rising out of the ashes like the phoenix. Inhale back to centre and exhale to the other side.
- Standing Heart opening Arch/Anahatasana to Standing Forward Fold/Padangusthasana, three times.
- Downward Dog, peddling the feet, bending one knee then the other. Inhale lift the right leg up and back and lift the right hip, draping the right foot behind. Students should feel an opening through the hip flexor region. Release the right leg down and do the same with the left leg.
- Slowly lower to Chaturanga Dandasana
- Seated Head to Knee/Janu Sirsasana Variation
- Bound Angle/Baddha Konasana
- Neck Stretches with Shoulder Shrugs

Body of Class:
Sohum Mindfulness Practice: One of the most accessible ways to practice **Swadhyaya** (self-study) is through mindfulness. When the mind becomes quiet and the breath steady, we create space to observe our thoughts, patterns, and inner dialogue. **Japa**, the repetition of a sound, word, or phrase, helps to focus the mind in the present moment. Through this focused awareness, we can access intuition, inner wisdom, and respond to the deeper questions of the heart.

Practice Instructions:
- **Set Up Your Space**
  - Find a comfortable seated position.
  - Place in front of you an item that inspires a sense of peace and comfort. If you do not have a physical item, visualize one in your mind's eye.
- **Begin with Fall-Out Breaths**
  - Take several Fall-Out Breaths: inhale through the nose and exhale through the mouth with a soft sigh.
  - Allow the outer body to relax while maintaining an upright posture, with the head aligned over the spine.
- **Hand Placement (Mudra)**

- o Bring your hands into **Jnana Mudra**: touch the pads of the forefinger and thumb together.
  - o Rest the hands on the thighs or knees.
  - o Palms facing **up**: invites expanded awareness.
  - o Palms facing **down**: encourages inward focus and quieting of the mind.
- **Mantra Practice (Japa)**
  - o Soften your gaze on the object in front of you (or your imagined item).
  - o With each breath cycle:
  - o Inhale while mentally or softly saying **"So"** *(I am)*.
  - o Exhale while saying **"Hum"** *(That)*.
  - o The mantra **Sohum** reflects the understanding: *I am that — I am part of the universal wisdom and connected to the vast, expansive energy that links all beings through breath.*
- **Continue for 5–7 minutes**
  - o Maintain a steady, smooth breath.
  - o Keep the spine tall and the belly soft as you continue the repetition.
- **Closing the Practice**
  - o Bring your hands to the heart center in **Anjali Mudra** (prayer position).
  - o Acknowledge the mantra, **Sohum**, and the item that supported your practice.

Closing:
- Lie down and settle into Savasana, applying eye pillows if available.
- Invite students to continue to quietly recite Sohum during their time of rest.
- Journal about this focusing experience.

Reflection/Conclusion

Learning about ourselves and our interconnectedness brings peace and wellness to our relationships. If everyone were to take time to be mindfully still, can you imagine how it would change the way people interact? Open the floor to discussion.

OMwork

Create a home practice zone by finding a low traffic spot in your house that you can claim as your own space. On a shelf (or cover a box with a piece of cloth), create an altar where you can put the item you brought into class, photos of inspiring leaders, loved ones (including yourself), quotes, flowers, bells etc. This unique space is yours to design in the way you wish that will inspire your practice and serve as a reminder of the well of knowledge that resides within.
*Students can take photos or a video of this space and submit it for assessment.

OMwork Material

Handout on Self-Reflection/Swadhyaya

The Importance of Self-Reflection

Self-reflection can be a challenging practice for many. It calls for personal accountability, which often feels harder than the more instinctive response of blaming others—or even ourselves. Because of this, self-reflection requires emotional intelligence. While our society tends to value IQ (intelligence quotient), EQ, or emotional intelligence, is frequently underestimated or overlooked.

Think of someone who is intellectually brilliant but has low emotional or social intelligence. They may excel academically and professionally, yet struggle in their personal relationships because they're unaware of how their behavior affects others. They might act in ways that don't align with their values—or worse, may lack awareness of their values or moral principles altogether.

True personal growth, however, depends on honest self-reflection and a willingness to take responsibility for our actions, especially when we err. Instead of drowning in shame or blame, we recognize that life is a series of lessons. The practice of *Swadhyaya*—self-study—helps us adjust our course with each experience as we strive to become the person we aspire to be.

These are the foundations of emotional and social intelligence. Without them, one might succeed in some areas but struggle deeply in relationships and matters of the heart.

You deserve the best life has to offer, and self-reflection nurtures essential relational skills like resolving conflicts, building meaningful connections, and growing emotionally.

As you practice self-reflection, consider asking yourself:
- What values matter most to me?
- What qualities do I seek in new friendships?
- How do I treat myself when I make mistakes?
- What does it mean to take responsibility for myself without harsh judgment?
- What does self-love mean to me?
- What actions show self-love, and why is it important?
- What triggers my social anxiety?
- What fears or worries do I carry?
- What kind of person do I want to become?
- How can self-reflection guide me toward becoming that person?

Swadhyaya invites us to listen to our deepest desires and follow the guidance of our hearts. #FollowYourHeart!

Daily Lesson Plan #26:
Self-Study/Swadhyaya and Sacred Texts

Intention/Objective
Students will examine various traditional texts and select an excerpt that inspires their journey.
Teaching Resource Material
Art supplies with craft paper.
Review/Introduction
There is much to learn about the different traditions and today we are going to research the main texts and choose a segment from one that awakens our desire to learn more.
Lesson

Centering:
- Self-reflection/Swadhyaya Affirmation- When I learn about the spirit of life, I better understand myself and my purpose.

Body of Class:
- Note: Please ensure that research is of a positive, helpful manner and that no content involves violence or harm to oneself or others.
- Browse through several sacred texts, such as:
- Braiding Sweetgrass
- The Bible
- The Bhagavad Gita
- The Yoga Sutras
- The Qur'an
- The Torah
- The Tao te Ching
- The Dhammapada
- Course in Miracles
- Your own choice
- Write a half page quote or wisdom teaching from one text on craft paper. Decorate it with images or drawings. Present it to the class, explaining why it interests you and put it on the classroom wall for the remainder of the term.

Closing:
- Students can share their reflections in their journal or in an open discussion on their peers' chosen pieces.
- **Affirmation**: When I learn about the spirit of life, I better understand myself and my purpose.

Reflection/Conclusion

- There are many gems of wisdom to be gleaned from each tradition, and there is a common thread running through each, which is the energy of creation that breathes life into each one of us.
- **Final Quote**: "Thou shalt not judge, because thou hast messed up in the past also."

OMwork

- Take the excerpt you chose from the text that inspires insight and report on it through a one-page written reflection.
- Choose an asana that represents the excerpt you chose.
- Explain why you chose this asana and how it relates to Swadhyaya, your personal growth.

Daily Lesson Plan #27:
Belief in love/Ishvara Pranidhana

Intention/Objective
Students will explore what it means to live with an awareness and belief in love.
Review/Introduction
<ul><li>Just as Ahimsa is the most important Yama, Belief in Love/Ishvara Pranidhana is the most important Niyama. As we practice this Niyama, all the others fall into place.</li><li>This Niyama encourages us to focus on the quality of our thoughts and actions, to contribute to this invisible, yet powerful stream of love.</li><li>Discuss the word surrender; to yield, stop trying to fix and let it flow. When we stop trying to fix ourselves, we can accept our own goodness. We are like one wave in the vast ocean of the whole of life, we are all essential components of the big picture. When we practice Ishvara Pranidhana, we learn to surrender to the uncertainties of life by trusting the process.</li><li>**Affirmation for Ishvara Pranidhana**-I surrender to the Love Intelligence that is around me and within me, supporting me always.</li></ul>
Lesson

Centering:
- Many traditions believe there are two main emotions: fear and love. When we are not acting with love, we are acting from fear.
- Fear constricts our energy and dampens our spirits. We act out of fear when we relate to others through combat, conflict or criticism.
- How do you feel when you are in fear?
- What situations instill fear? (fear of failure, looking stupid, criticism, basic needs threatened etc). Is there an asana that demonstrates this natural feeling?
- Love, on the other hand, is expansive, creative, playful and all-embracing.
- We act of love when we relate to others through connection, calmness and curiosity.
- How do you feel when you are in the presence of love?
- What situations awaken love within you? (time with a grandparent, good friends, yoga practice etc).
- Is there an asana that demonstrates this high frequency feeling?

Body of Class:
- Option 1: Compile the students' asanas that represent love and do these for your asana practice.
- Option 2: Move through the following Heart Opening Movement Class:
- Hands overlapping at the heart and circling over the upper chest to connect to this powerful center of love
- Neck stretches
- Shoulder rotations
- Tricep stretch, switch sides
- Posterior deltoid stretch (arm reaches across in front of chest)
- Eagle arms/Garudasana
- Downward Dog to Table to Cat/Cow three times, repeat the whole cycle three times.
- Dolphin/Pincha Mayurasana Prep, elbows to the floor with a block between the web of the hands and pressed against the wall. Inhale and lift the right leg up and exhale lower it, same on the other side.
- Child's/Balasana, breathe in love, breathe out love
- Powerful/Utkatasana to Yoga Mudra three times
- Dancer/Natarajasana

Daily Lesson Plan #27: Belief in love/Ishvara Pranidhana

- Partner asana: Bow/Dhanurasana Prep - partner A stands with arms open out to the sides and partner B stands behind, with hands on their forearms, drawing the arms toward each other behind. Switch roles.
- Partner Dhanurasana: Partner A lies on belly and enters the Bow, while partner B straddles partner A's waist and sits on the soles of their feet. Partner B then gently pulls partner A's shoulders back to help open the chest.

Closing:
- Pigeon/Eka Pada Raja Kapotasana: lift torso perpendicular to the floor first to open the heart, then lower to Sleeping Pigeon or any variation of their choice.
- Legs up the wall/Viparita Karani. As you relax, allow whatever you're clinging to gently release and drift away, making space for the goodness, beauty and love that exists all around you.

Reflection/Conclusion

- In Sukhasana/Easy or Virasana/Hero, bring hands to heart and keep them about 3 inches away from one another.
- Can you palpate the energy of your heart centre within your hands?
- Pulse the hands with each breath to massage this ball of energy, letting it expand within your awareness. Think of someone who's done amazing things with the power of their love as you charge your heart energy.
- With hands in Anjali Mudra, send this energy out with your breath and hands from the heart, circling back to your heart, three times.

OMwork

- Where can you be a leader in bringing more love to the world? (Start with yourself, then move to your friends and family). #FollowyourHeart
- Choose a song that reflects one of the Niyamas and bring it to class the next day.

OMwork Material

- Students can be given a section of clay to create an art piece that reflects this Niyama.
- These art forms can be displayed in the classroom.

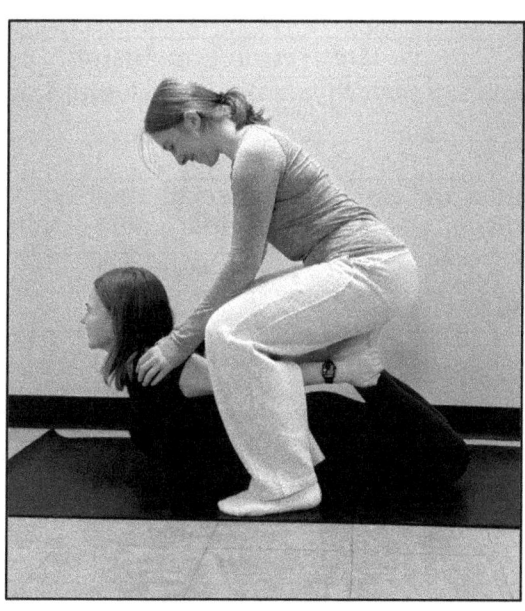

Daily Lesson Plan #28: Review of Niyamas

Intention/Objective
To summarize and solidify the message of the Niyamas.
Review/Introduction
Review the definition of each Niyama and speak out their affirmations together.
Lesson
Centering: • Come to a seated position and invite students to recall the five Niyamas and their translation. • Trace the other hand and title each digit with a Niyama. Keep both hands with the Yamas and Niyamas at the front of your mats as you practice. **Body of Class:** • Sun Salutation A, five times to symbolize the Niyamas, reading the affirmation for each at the beginning of the Salutation. • Have each student **choose one posture** from the 50 foundational asanas that reflects one Niyama and do that individually. • Shoulder Pressing Arm Balance/Bhujapidasana with hands/hastas on blocks or on the floor, with each finger representing the Yamas and Niyamas. • Divide the class into groups of four or five. Assign a Niyama to each group and give them time to create a sequence of five asanas that reflect their assigned Niyama (for example, Swadhyaya might look like Mountain to Camel, to Downward Dog to Child's to Hero). Each group can present their asanas to the class, with the music of their choosing. **Closing:** • Full Yogic Breathing in **Easy Asana/Sukhasana** or **Relaxation/Savasana**, while listening to one of the selected songs from the asana activity.
Reflection/Conclusion
In a circle, have the students say each Niyama in English and Sanskrit and finish with the sound of OM.
OMwork
Journal entry to be submitted and assessed: Reflect on the Niyama that you would like to focus on for the next week. How will you make this principle a part of your daily life?
OMwork Material
The Yamas and Niyamas in Review

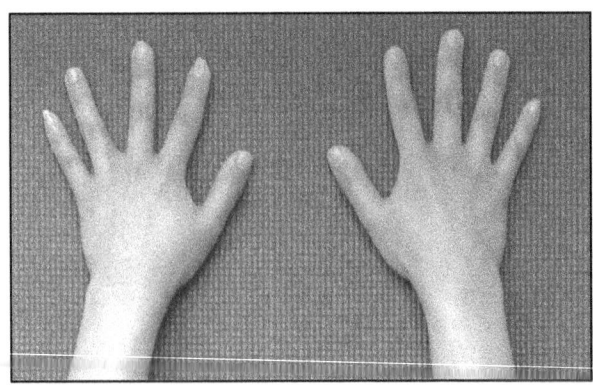

Daily Lesson Plan #28:
Review of Niyamas

The First Two Limbs in Review (20 points)

1. How are the Yamas and Niyamas different from the Ten Commandments?
(1 Pt)
- There is no religious godhead behind them.

2. What is the main focus of the Yamas?
(1 Pt)
- How to treat others respectfully.

3. What is the main purpose of the Niyamas?
(1 Pt)
- How to treat ourselves respectfully.

Yamas

4. In your own words, describe the meaning of Ahimsa.
(1 Pt)
- Kindness.

5. By practicing Satya, we can live with more _____.
(1 Pt)
- Integrity, freedom, self-love (accept any relevant answer).

6. Through the practice of Asteya, we move from scarcity and disbelief to creating _____ and _____.
(2 Pts)
- Financial stability, abundance, and confidence in our ability to fulfill our own dreams.

7. Give two examples of how you can apply Brahmacharya to your asana practice.
(2 Pts)
- Honoring your growing edge; turning your phone off (or minimizing distractions).

8. Which part of the breath (inhalation, retention, or exhalation) best relates to the practice of Aparigraha? Why?
(1 Pt)
- The exhalation, because it helps us let go of hoarding or attachment.

Take three deep breaths now, focusing on the exhalation.

Niyamas

9. What is one benefit of practicing Saucha?
(1 Pt)
- Fewer regrets because we become more mindful of what we say and do; less drama and conflict.

10. List two industries that promote anti-Santosha by creating feelings of self-hatred, longing, or jealousy.
(2 Pts)
- Fashion, beauty, entertainment, social media.

11. Reflect on the Niyama of Tapas. How might regular practice improve two aspects of your life?
(2 Pts)
- Developing self-discipline in maintaining a regular exercise routine, sleep schedule, or completing homework.

Daily Lesson Plan #28:
Review of Niyamas

12. What are three things you have discovered about yourself through the practice of Swadhyaya?
(3 Pts)
- Examples: I work too much; I have social anxieties; I resist self-reflection due to shame.

13. Why do you think the ancient yogis identified Ishvara Pranidhana as the most important of all the Niyamas?
(2 Pts)
- Trusting life helps to alleviate anxiety and deepens our faith in goodness.

Daily Lesson Plan #29:
The Mindful Limbs of Raja Yoga

Intention/Objective
<ul><li>So far, we've focused on the first four limbs of Raja Yoga, which include the Five Yamas, the Five Niyamas, Asanas/postures and Pranayama/breathwork.</li><li>Let's spend this class exploring the subtler practices of mindful awareness and stilling the activity between the ears.</li><li>Although these practices were developed 5,000 years ago, with the dawn of the digital age, they've become more necessary than ever.</li></ul>
Teacher Resource Material
Soft music, cushions or yoga mats
Introduction/Review
"The ability to focus is becoming the scarcest commodity of the 21st century. Focus is like a mental muscle: through deliberate training, you can strengthen your focus and expand your mental capacity." ~ Cal Newport, Deep Work <ul><li>In an ancient yogic legend, there is a story of a great warrior. When the other warriors were asked what they saw when viewing a target in a tree, they said the branches, the leaves, the landscape etc. This warrior, however, saw just one thing; the center of his target, which reflected his astonishing ability to concentrate on his goal.</li><li>Industries are profiting on our attention, and yet attention is one of the top qualities we need to fulfill our dreams and create a life we love.</li></ul> Note to Teacher: <ul><li>Before embarking on a mindfulness practice, it is important for students to realize that mindfulness is not about emptying the mind, as this is a very rare and challenging accomplishment. Instead, the intent is to become a witness who watches the stream of thoughts without engaging them. Mindfulness is also about fully absorbing yourself in the moment and noticing every detail of it.</li><li>This practice involves the limbs of **Pratyahara**, or withdrawal of the senses from the outside world, **Dharana**, concentration on the present, with attempts to reach **Dhyana**, prolonged concentration.</li><li>If there is a great deal of external sounds or if your student population is easily distracted, you can play soft music, like Nada Himalayan by Deuter, as you read the script.</li></ul>
Lesson
Centering: See handout on Dopamine versus Oxytocin to open discussion. **Body of Class:** The following script can be read aloud by the teacher: <ul><li>Come to a seated position, either in a chair, on your yoga mat or if necessary, you can lean against the wall. If it is comfortable, you can sit in **Easy Asana (Sukhasana)** or Half Lotus (Ardha Padmasana). Bring your fingers into **Jnana Mudra** with forefingers and thumbs together—turn palms face down to feel grounded or turn the palms upward to increase your energy.</li><li>Roll the **shoulders back and down**, aligning the ears over the shoulders and the shoulders over the hips.</li></ul>

Daily Lesson Plan #29:
The Mindful Limbs of Raja Yoga

- Visualize a **string attached to the crown** of your head, attaching to each vertebra, extending down through your seat and connecting to the earth. Now imagine a puppet master tugging on the string, aligning your spine from your tailbone to your crown, and allowing energy to flow freely. Make any final adjustments to your sitting position before beginning our sitting mindfulness practice.
- Bring your attention to the breath as it enters through the nostrils, drifting down to the base of the lungs, gently pressing out on the walls of the belly. Feel the air leave your body, through the nostrils as well.
- Allow your **breath to become like a wave,** gently flowing in and out. As you continue with this breathing pattern, you as the witness, will notice that your mind wants to engage in the drama of thinking. When you observe yourself engaging in thinking, **label it 'thinking'** and return to home base—which is your breath. Focus on the breath entering through the nostrils, filling the belly and ribs and flowing back out again.
- Imagine yourself sitting on the **bank of a river**, watching leaves float by one by one. Each leaf symbolizes a thought that consumes our minds energy and attention. Just continue to watch these leaves float by, letting **thoughts come and go**. When you are tempted to pick one up and engage in the flurry of thinking, return to your breath awareness, smoothly **breathing in and breathing out.**
- Note for teacher: After two minutes of mindful breathing in silence, read the following:
  - As you sit here, your mind may begin to wander. Label it thinking and come back to your breathing until you become one with the breath, flowing in and out.
- **Note to Teacher**: This whole process will take approximately 15 minutes. When you are done, ring a practice bell (or find a bell on an app) and gently draw the student's attention back to the classroom.

Closing:
See handout: Debrief by discussing answers to the following questions:
- Have you practiced mindfulness before?
- Was it frustrating or boring?
- Was it relaxing or enjoyable?
- How did you react to your experiences? (with impatience or with kindness?)
- Can you see the benefit of doing this practice regularly?
- What might change in your life if you started a practice?

OMwork

- Research the physical and mental benefits of a mindfulness practice and bring your findings to the next class to be discussed.
- Write a reflection on this quote and how it applies to your life:
- "You must have a clear mind if you want to realize the Self. Unless the mind casts away desires, cravings, worries, pride, lust - it cannot enter the domain of peace." Dr. Sivananda

Omwork Material

Handouts: Dopamine versus Oxytocin and
Mindfulness Journal Reflection

Dopamine versus Oxytocin

"If we're spending most of our lives in the virtual world, we're not really living at all." ~ Dr. Carrion

We're living in a tech-obsessed world that's constantly feeding our brains dopamine—and it's messing with our mood.

Dopamine is the brain chemical that gives us a quick rush of pleasure. Back in the day, it only spiked when we did something essential—like finding food or discovering something new. Now? Every notification, like, or scroll on our phone gives us another hit.

Because of this nonstop stimulation, we're hooked on screens—and when we're not on them, we feel irritable, anxious, or bored. This is one of the biggest reasons so many people feel disconnected and overwhelmed.

Here's the catch: the more we chase dopamine, the less we get of another important brain chemical—**oxytocin**. Oxytocin builds trust, connection, and calm. It's what we feel during a meaningful hug, a deep talk, or when we laugh with friends.

Low oxytocin levels are linked to anxiety, stress, and restlessness—exactly what so many of us are struggling with right now.

So how do we fix it? We start by choosing connection over constant stimulation.

That means:
- More **face-to-face** conversations
- **Real hugs** and handshakes
- **Listening** without distractions
- Giving genuine **compliments**
- Asking deep, thoughtful **questions**

The more we do these things, the more oxytocin we build—and the better we feel.

Let's create more phone-free moments filled with presence, connection, and calm. Your oxytocin oasis is waiting.

Mindfulness Journal Reflection

Take a few quiet moments to reflect on your experiences with mindfulness. Use the questions below to guide your journaling. There are no right or wrong answers—just be honest with yourself.

1. **Have you ever practiced mindfulness before?** If yes, describe when and how.
2. **What was that experience like for you?** Did you find it calming, frustrating, boring, or something else?
3. **Did you enjoy the experience?** What parts felt good or helpful? What didn't?
4. **How did you treat yourself during the practice?** Were you patient and gentle, or did you feel frustrated or critical?
5. **Can you see any benefits to practicing mindfulness regularly?** What might those benefits be for your body, mind, or emotions?
6. **If you committed to a consistent mindfulness practice, what changes could you imagine happening in your life?** Think about how it might affect your stress levels, focus, relationships, or sense of self.

Daily Lesson Plan #30:
The Eight Limbs Creative Art Piece

Intention/Objective
Students will design an art piece in partners, or in small groups, that depict the Eight Limbs of Raja Yoga.
Review/Introduction

We've explored the first seven limbs of yoga—now we arrive at the eighth: **Samadhi**.
    Samadhi is often described as a state of **higher awareness** or **deep inner bliss**. It's that feeling of complete alignment—when you just know you're in the right place at the right time. You might experience it when your heart overflows with love for someone special, when you witness an act of profound kindness, or when you feel so at peace that you gently drift into restful sleep.
    It's not something we chase, but something we naturally move toward through consistent practice and presence.
 	
"The most beautiful thing we can experience is the mysterious. It is the source of all true art and science." — Albert Einstein

Lesson
Let's bring the spirit of Samadhi—that feeling of deep peace, connection, and purpose—into our group activity.<ul><li>Your task is to create an **art piece** that reflects the **Eight Limbs of Yoga**. You can choose to work individually, in pairs, or as a full class. How you express the eight limbs is entirely up to you—be creative and let your ideas flow.</li><li>Here are a few examples to spark inspiration:<ul><li>Some students have painted a tree on a classroom or hallway wall, naming each branch after one of the Eight Limbs.</li><li>Others have designed a mandala on the double doors to the yoga studio, weaving the limbs into the design.</li><li>You might write a song, choreograph a movement piece, create a poem, or paint on canvas.</li></ul></li><li>Your creation can be anything (within reason!) that thoughtfully represents the Eight Limbs as a path of human development. This is your chance to express how these teachings live and breathe in your life—through color, shape, words, or sound, by painting, drawing, writing poetry, composing music, creating movement or any other artistic expression.</li></ul>**Centering:**<ul><li>Begin by flowing together in a Namaskar to harmonize the class's intent and energy.</li></ul>**Body of Class:**<ul><li>Collectively create a plan with the class that everyone is happy with.</li><li>Provide craft supplies and get to work.</li></ul>**Closing:**<ul><li>Savasana with lower legs on the seat of chairs to alleviate any back strain from the crafting.</li><li>Quote: *"When the channels of the body and mind are clear, creativity flows like breath—effortless, pure, and deeply connected to spirit."* Inspired by yogic teachings</li></ul>**Reflection/Conclusion:**<ul><li>Take a group photo of the art piece (s).</li></ul>

Daily Lesson Plan #30:
The Eight Limbs Creative Art Piece

OMwork
• Reflect on the creative artwork in your journal. • Send a photo and a description to the student counsel so they can share it with the school.

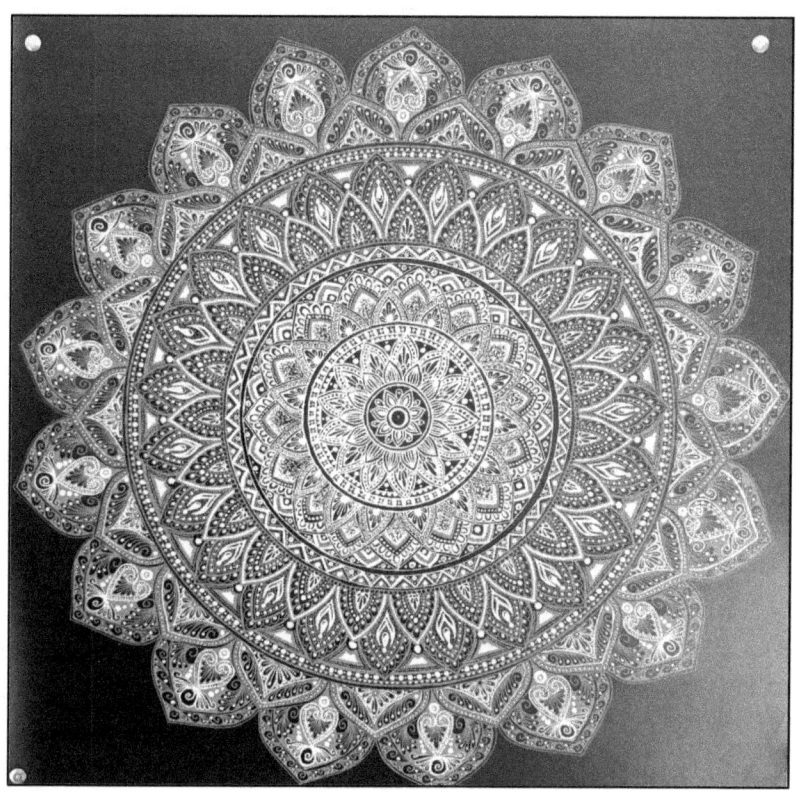

This is a mandala that the authors daughter, Bella, created during COVID at the age of 12.

Daily Lesson Plan #31: Letting Go Ritual

Intention/Objective
In this class, students will focus on releasing the suffering that's preventing them from being their best self, focusing on what's within their control.
Review/Introduction
<ul><li>In Yoga there is a term called **Samskaras**, which are habit patterns of the mind, stemming from past experiences and memories. In modern psychology this is referred to as **cognitive distortions or thinking errors**. These samskaras tend to be created at a very young age.</li><li>Not knowing there is another way of thinking, many people replay these patterns or beliefs over and over for the rest of their lives, like a broken record. These thought patterns are often unhealthy and **keep us stuck in negative** thinking and feeling (fear, unworthiness, resentment).</li><li>For example: As a child, Timmy was told he was a crappy singer and advised to lip sync the words in the Christmas concert. From that day forward, he experiences great anxiety whenever he finds himself in a situation that involves singing. Was Timmy a terrible singer? No, but that choir director's opinion dampened his vocal confidence for the rest of his life!</li></ul>
Lesson
Centering:<ul><li>In partners, discuss your perspective on samskaras or limiting beliefs and how they influence people's lives. Think of examples in your friend group or family.</li><li>On a piece of paper, **record a thinking error** or limiting belief that replays in your mind. Write down all the ways it's affected you and influenced your choices.</li><li>Now reflect on what your life would look like if you were able to grow out of that negative story. Describe what your life would look like if you were free of this negative pattern.</li><li>Write on another sheet of paper "**Today I let go of**…", a Samskaras or destructive thought pattern that you are ready to release and move beyond. Fold it and place it by your mat.</li><li>*Note: A Smudge Ceremony outdoors is helpful for cleansing old energy.</li></ul>**Body of Class:**<ul><li>Let's explore asanas that shake up our current cellular reality.</li><li>**Full body shake**, starting with the hands, shoulders, head, bouncing in the knees, letting your body shake it out.</li><li>Stand up and **gather energy** with your arms overhead and exhale, with palms down, lower your hands down your front body, sweeping your energy field from head to toe.</li><li>**Laughter Yoga**: Close your eyes and awaken the feeling inside that would accompany the freedom from negative self-talk, if you truly knew that you weren't broken, but that you are gifted and worthy of love. Bring that feeling into the next activity.</li><li>Inhale arms overhead and exhale fold forward hanging the head and arms. On the exhale as you fold forward, laugh your way down to hanging your head. Let it all out and keep encouraging the laughter from the belly. If they are having a hard time, tell a silly story or joke to get things rolling, like: "How do squirrel's close a yoga class? NUTmaste!"</li><li>They can also sound out the vowels like "Hahaha, Heeheehee…" or make silly faces.</li><li>There are also recordings of laughing babies on YouTube to assist in the flow!</li><li>Hopefully the class will continue the momentum, with the laughter becoming more spontaneous.</li><li>Be warned, people in the halls will likely stop and smile or even join in. Imagine the power of merging a few classes together in a session of laughter Yoga?</li><li>Quote to close laughter session: "**Laughter is the same in all languages.**"</li></ul>

- **Table/Bharmanasana** with cat/cow, inhaling into cat and exhaling into cow with Lion's Breath.
- **Beetle on its back:** see Elementary posters. Lie on your back and lift arms and legs up like a beetle trying to flip over. Begin to shake the hands and then the feet, put it altogether and shake every limb harder and harder. Tuck knees to chest when finished and breathe deeply. Think of the Samskara you are releasing and focus on shaking it out of your body in the next round.
- Do Beetle on its back a second time.
- **Supine Leg Lifts:** start on your back with legs up, with palms facing down under sacrum. Lower and lift one leg at a time for ten times. To further engage the core, lift your head.
- Scale Asana/Lolasana on blocks to create tapas and feel the lightness of letting go.

Closing:
- Restorative asana of your choice: Legs up the wall/Viparita Karani, Child's/Balasana or Relaxation/Savasana.
- We are what we think about, and yoga teaches us that we can purge the unproductive thoughts from our awareness and choose more helpful, uplifting ones. By letting go of past scars (and samskaras), we can chart our own course in life.

Reflection/Conclusion

As you leave the room, tear up your sheet of paper with your limiting belief on it and throw it in the paper recycling bin.

OMwork

Write yourself a letter, from the older, wiser, kinder self within you. Let this letter remind you of your worthiness and help you to believe in your dreams. Add this to your wellness portfolio.

Sample Letter to Your Current Self

Dear _____,

You are so much stronger than you realize. I know that life seems like the challenges will never end. But you will get through this—and not just get through it but grow because of it.

You are learning, every single day, even if it doesn't always feel like progress. Those moments of doubt, fear, and frustration? They are part of your journey, shaping you into the resilient, compassionate person you're destined to become.

Remember to be gentle with yourself. You don't have to have all the answers today. It's okay to take your time, to rest, to ask for help. Your worth is not measured by your productivity or perfection, but by your willingness to keep going.

Hold on to your dreams, even when they seem distant. Keep nurturing your creativity, your curiosity, and your kindness. These qualities will light your path when times are dark.

You are so loved—not just by others, but by yourself. And as you grow older, I hope you see yourself through my eyes: full of potential, courage, and endless possibility.

Keep believing in yourself, because I'm rooting for you every step of the way.

With love and hope,
Your Older Self

Daily Lesson Plan #32: Intention Setting 1

Intention/Objective
This class will assist students in gaining clarity on what their passion and life purpose are.
Review/Introduction
<ul><li>To fulfill your deepest dreams, you must release the need for approval from others.</li><li>Through our practice, the noise of the outside world fades, and we begin to reconnect with our truest nature and most heartfelt desires.</li><li>We come to see that we are the architects of our lives—what we consistently focus on, we amplify and attract.</li><li>Often, who we are today is the outcome of beliefs we held three, six, or even twelve months ago.</li><li>Our physical reality is frequently a reflection of what's happening within our minds.</li><li>Let's take a few moments to pause, reflect, and ask ourselves: **What do I truly want from life?**</li></ul>**Note:** This reflection is not a competition for wealth or status. It's an invitation to clarify your unique gifts and explore how you might offer them to the world in meaningful, authentic ways. See Ego versus the Self handout for Omwork.
Lesson
Intention setting practice (to soft music):<ul><li>Begin by lying back on your mat, settling into a comfortable and restful position.</li><li>Make a quiet commitment to remain present throughout this experience, resisting the temptation to drift off to sleep.</li><li>Gently observe your breath, allowing it to slow and deepen. Let this steady rhythm bring a wave of calm into your body. Soften the muscles of your face, your scalp, your neck and throat. Release tension in your chest and belly, allowing your pelvic floor to relax. Let go through your legs, calves, and feet—until your entire body is resting in a deep state of relaxation.</li><li>Exhale with a sigh a few times to anchor this feeling of release.</li><li>With your breath now natural and easy, visualize yourself standing at the edge of a woodland path.</li><li>Step forward onto the trail, surrounded by tall trees, dappled light, and the sounds of nature. As you walk, take in the beauty around you—the wildflowers, the scent of fresh earth, the soft rustle of leaves.</li><li>Turning a gentle corner, you encounter your first obstacle. This obstacle represents a limiting belief you've been holding about yourself.</li><li>Name it. Recognize it for what it is.</li><li>Ask yourself: **What small step could I take to begin letting this go?**</li><li>(Pause for reflection.)</li><li>As this obstacle dissolves, you continue along the path with renewed strength. The air begins to shift with the scent of salt, and you breathe in deeply.</li><li>Up ahead, another challenge appears—another limiting belief or perception.</li><li>Identify it. Acknowledge its presence.</li><li>Ask yourself: **How do I choose to move beyond this now?**</li><li>(Pause for reflection.)</li><li>You feel yourself growing lighter and freer with every step.</li><li>The forest opens, and you arrive at a serene beach where the ocean meets the shore.</li><li>Slip off your shoes and feel the warm, soft sand beneath your feet.</li><li>Let the gentle waves and wide-open sky welcome you.</li></ul>

Daily Lesson Plan #32:
Intention Setting 1

- Find a quiet place to rest—perhaps lying in the sun or tucked under the shade of a tree branch. Allow your heart to open and your mind to wander.
- Invite your deepest desires to rise gently to the surface.
- The vast blue sky reminds you: in the realm of creativity, there are no limits.
- Let yourself dream—freely, boldly, joyfully—of what you love and how you long to live.
- Take two minutes for quiet reflection.
- It's now time to begin your return journey.
- Slowly, gently, imagine yourself rising and walking back along the forest trail.
- As you pass the places where your old obstacles once stood, smile—notice how easily you step over them now.
- With every breath, feel your dreams taking deeper root in your being.
- You arrive back at the place where your journey began—renewed, inspired, and filled with gratitude for the insights you've gained.
- Slowly begin to deepen your breathing and stretch your arms overhead, making your body as long as possible. Tuck your right knee into your chest and hold for a few breaths. Guide the knee across the midline of the body with the left hand, stretching the right arm out or up to complete the twisting action through the spine. If possible, straighten the right leg and hold the foot with the left hand.
- After five breaths, return to centre, tuck knee to chest and release the right leg. Switch sides.
- With palms down, slide hands beneath the buttocks, palms down and lift into Fish/Matsyasana for five or so breaths, letting the heart blossom. Gradually release out of the Fish.
- Turn your head from side to side, freeing the neck.
- Gently roll over and rise to seated and then fold forward into Seated Forward Fold/Paschimottanasana or Bound Angle/Baddha Konasana for five to ten breaths.
- Rise to sitting and centre your energy for a moment in silence.
- Discuss in small groups what occurred on the journey and what you discovered.
- Read quote: *"When you are inspired by some greater purpose, some extraordinary project, all your thoughts break their bonds, your mind transcends limitations, your consciousness expands in every direction, and you find yourself in a new and wonderful world. Dormant forces and talents become alive, and you discover yourself to be a greater person than you ever dreamed yourself to be."* ~Patanjali
- "Love to" List: As a class, at the top of a clean sheet of paper or in your journal, write a "Love To" List. For three straight minutes, as fast as you can, write down all the things you love. Include things that feed your senses, like bubble baths, or flowers, and things you loved to do as a child.
- When the time is up, read through your list and add any remaining items that you missed.
- Share with a partner some of your responses.
- Did anything surprise you on your list?
- How can you incorporate these items that you love into your daily life?
- How will this list inform your choices for the future?

Closing:
"Thoughts become things, so choose the good ones!"- Mike Dooley

Reflection/Conclusion

In order to see different results in our lives, we must do different things and think in different ways.

OMwork

- Journal about your guided visualization.
- Continue to expand your "Love To" List.
- For our next class, bring in magazines or search online for photos that reflect your personal interests and future dreams.

Daily Lesson Plan #32:
Intention Setting 1

OMwork Material
Watch an inspiring documentary or movie on a person who's defied the odds, like 'Unstoppable', a documentary about the one-legged wrestling champ, Anthony Robles.

Today, I'll see my life as if it's brand new

Today, I'll see the world like it's brand new.
The way the clouds float across the open sky,
How music hits differently when I'm really listening,
And how someone's laugh can change a whole moment.

Today, I'll let myself experience everything fully,
The intricate details of a loved one's face,
The joy of other's successes,
The space between thoughts.
Today, I won't take anything for granted.
I'll silence my phone and hear the sounds of nature.
I'll listen to a friend a little longer.
I'll let myself daydream and envision what's possible.

Today, I'll imagine something bold,
For myself,
For the people I care about,
For a world that could be better, kinder, more authentic.

Today, I'll stretch further than I think I can.
I'll stay grounded in who I truly am.
I'll dream out loud,
And choose to believe that I matter.

Today, I'll see my life as if it's brand new.

Daily Lesson Plan #33: Intention Setting 2

Intention/Objective
Students will explore their dreams by creating visual representations of them.
Teaching Resource Material
<ul><li>Art supplies for creating collages: Poster paper, scissors, glue/tape, magazines or printed online images.</li><li>Wheel of life Handout</li></ul>
Review/Introduction
<ul><li>In the last class we worked to dissolve the obstacles in the way of our best life and gained clarity on things we love.</li><li>In small groups, discuss your new awareness of the obstacles that were in your life and the action steps you are taking to move you forward.</li><li>Today we'll look at the various components of our lives and assess the areas that we wish to enhance.</li></ul>
Lesson
Centering:<ul><li>Sun Breaths</li><li>Awaken creative energy by flowing through Sun Salutations to music</li></ul>**Body of Class:**<ul><li>Have students fill out the wheel of life by drawing a line across each pie to indicate their degree of satisfaction with each area of life. Zero fulfillment is in the very center of the pie and ten is out at the periphery. Now color in the space from zero to the number chosen to clearly illustrate how well they're living a "Love To" life.</li><li>Take one area of your life that you'd like to focus on and write that on the top of a blank page.</li><li>Envision the result, with this section at a 10/10 and describe the details of this state.</li><li>Self-esteem and belief in ourselves are developed by doing estimable things.</li><li>List three achievable action steps to enhance this aspect of your wheel and propel you toward your best life. Perhaps it's as simple as joining a gym, starting your day with mindfulness, building a basic website or applying to volunteer etc.</li></ul>**Closing:**<ul><li>Collages - with poster paper, browse online or in magazines to find images that inspire you on this road to living your best life. The collage can focus on one area, or it can include all of them.</li><li>What words inspire you? Add them in between the graphics.</li><li>We can call these collages, or action boards, to remind us that we have to do more than just visualize, we must take daily action toward our goals.</li></ul>
Reflection/Conclusion
<ul><li>Choose what you want to create for your 'one wild and precious life.'</li><li>Dedicate yourself to it by doing something each day to support your vision.</li><li>An attitude of gratitude plays a major role in the manifestation process.</li><li>Have patience and be open to things unfolding in the way they're meant to.</li></ul>**Final Quote:** "You will get there when you are meant to get there and not one moment sooner. So relax, breathe, and be present to every stage of the journey." ~ Unknown

OMwork
<ul><li>Place your collage somewhere prominent in your life and reflect on it daily.</li><li>Whenever you look at your collage, take a moment to give thanks in advance for all your dreams coming true.</li><li>Choose a theme song (which the teacher can collect and compile for the class as an end of term present).</li></ul>
OMwork Material
Closing Quote: "Watch your thoughts, they become your words. Watch your words, they become your actions. Watch your actions, they become your habits. Watch your habits, they become your character. Watch your character, it becomes your destiny." ~ The Upanishads

The Wheel of Life

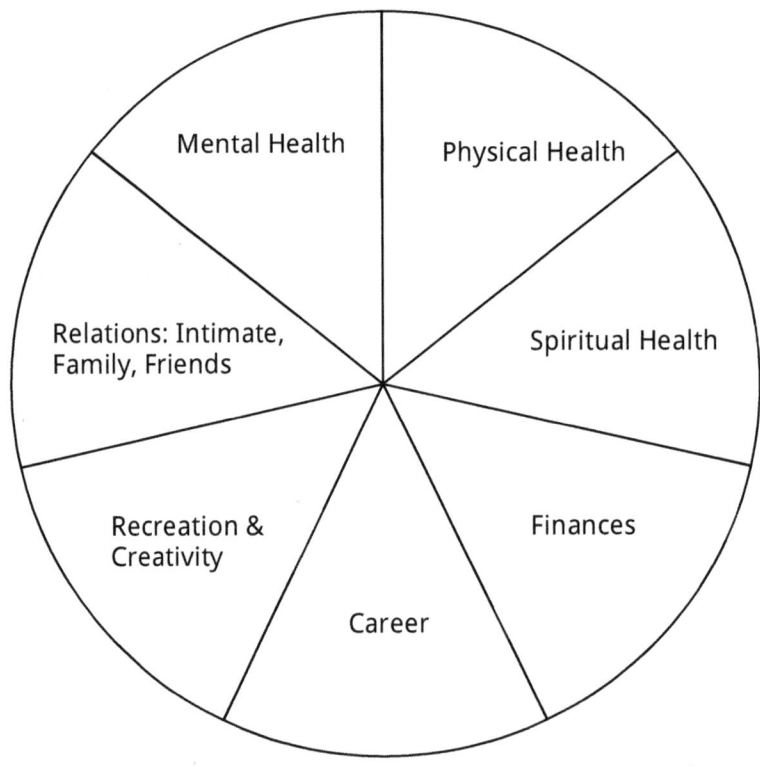

Daily Lesson Plan #34: Food as Medicine

Intention/Objective
This class is designed to draw awareness to how we nourish our body.
Teaching Resource Material
<ul><li>Article: The Yoga of Eating, one for each student.</li><li>Raisin Mindfulness Practice script or recording.</li></ul>
Review/Introduction
Review the koshas and the translation of the annamaya kosha (food layer, we are what we eat).
Lesson
<ul><li>Using the Secondary Yoga Posters (if available), invite students to partner up and choose three asanas each for warm-up, and lead your partner through them.</li><li>Read and discuss the article: The Yoga of Eating.</li><li>Discuss the difference between Sattvic, Rajasic and Tamasic foods, and note the readily available tamasic options in stores and restaurants.</li><li>Guide them through the Raisin Mindfulness Practice or play the recording of it.</li></ul>
Reflection/Conclusion
In class discussion, share your experience.
OMwork
<ul><li>Eat your next main meal the way you normally do and observe the way you feel afterward.</li><li>Eat another meal in silence, free of screens, and mindfully consume your food like you did the raisin.</li><li>Take a few minutes after your meal to sit quietly or go for a walk.</li><li>Note the differences.</li><li>Optional: Research the Ayurvedic model and follow up in the next class with a discussion on the results.</li><li>Note: Be sure to present Ayurveda as the approach to healthy eating that is most closely linked to the practice of yoga but not one that everyone needs to subscribe to.</li><li>Optional: Discuss food security, economic barriers to healthy eating and brainstorm strategies for eating well on a budget.</li><li>Bring a dish in for a potluck in your next yoga class.</li></ul>
OMwork Material
The Yoga of Eating Handout

Mindfulness Raisin Practice

Materials: organic raisins. Please encourage everyone to sanitize their hands before this exercise.

Give each participant a raisin and ask them to hold it in the palm of their hand. You can read the following script aloud or create your own version inspired by this guide.

For those beginning their mindfulness journey, it's helpful to remember the phrase: *"I do everything with a mind that lets go of distractions."*

Our minds tend to cling to thoughts, which then become sources of stress. The key is learning to let go, though this can be challenging. These restless thoughts are often called the "monkey mind," constantly jumping from one thing to another.

Daily Lesson Plan #34:
Food as Medicine

There's a well-known story from India about how monkeys are caught using a hollow log with a banana inside. When the monkey reaches into the log and grabs the banana, it tightly clenches its fist, making it impossible to pull out the banana. The monkey remains stuck, refusing to let go until the trapper captures it. The only way to be free is to release the banana. Our minds work similarly to the stubborn monkey, caught in cycles of repetitive thoughts and rumination.

This mindfulness exercise will help sharpen your attention on the present moment. Experiencing the here and now offers glimpses of freedom. There is a saying: *"The past is gone, the future is imagined, which is why the present moment is a gift."*

Now, look at the raisin in your hand. Notice its wrinkles, colors, and texture. You might see a small stem still attached—a reminder that this raisin was once connected to the vine, which grew from the earth, nourished by sunlight and soil.

Think about how this raisin reached you. After ripening on the vine, someone harvested it, placed it in a crate, and it traveled through a factory, warehouse, distributor, and finally arrived at the store where I bought it and brought it to you. Many people contributed their energy and care to bring this tiny fruit to your hand.

With this awareness, slowly roll the raisin between your fingers. Pause and notice the sensations—the feel of its folds and texture.

When you're ready, place the raisin on your tongue without biting. Feel it resting there and notice its texture. Gently press it between your front teeth and slowly pierce its skin, allowing the sweetness to spread in your mouth. Chew slowly at least 20 times, savoring the release of flavor with each bite. Chances are that this raisin has never tasted quite like this before.

When you feel ready, swallow the raisin. As it becomes part of you, remember that you are connected to the sun, the earth, and every person who played a role in bringing this raisin to your hand. Take a moment to appreciate this connection and your experience.

You have just practiced mindfulness—being fully present and focused on the simple act of eating.

OMwork: Bring a blessing or prayer your tradition recites before meals, or research one that resonates with you.

The Yoga of Eating

In Yoga, our physical body is often called the "food layer," because the substances we consume literally form the building blocks of our body. Our bodies are more than just the shape we see in the mirror—they are deeply connected to the ancient Earth, tracing back billions of years. Within every cell, we carry this innate intelligence. A yogic diet supports and nourishes this connection, helping us to flourish with vibrant health.

Brainstorm

What comes to mind when you think of a yogic diet?

A yogic diet is often described as a **Sattvic diet**. Here, the word "diet" means a way of eating, not necessarily eating less. The term *Sattvic* comes from Ayurveda, the ancient "Science of Life."

A Sattvic diet emphasizes food that is pure, clean, fresh, and wholesome. Fresh food means it is as close to its natural source as possible, allowing us to absorb not only nutrients but also the vital life energy of the food.

What do you think that means?

(Ideas might include eating local, organic, and recently harvested foods.)

Which foods wouldn't fit into this category?

(Tamasic foods such as canned, frozen, processed, or stale items.)
  Ayurveda also suggests eating with your hands. Handling food directly creates an energetic connection even before it touches your lips. Can you think of cultures that traditionally eat with their hands?
  Because of this, ancient healers advised that those preparing food should be in a calm and peaceful state.
  In Yoga, every step of eating—from preparation to consumption—is seen as part of the digestive process. So, a Sattvic diet involves not just what we eat, but how we eat. Eating in a calm environment and eating slowly—chewing thoroughly—helps the body digest more easily. This practice encourages us not only to savor the flavors and textures but also to appreciate the energy of the people who prepared the food and those we share the meal with.
  When we talk about savoring a meal, it means being fully present and aware of the senses. What habits do you notice that pull your attention away from truly enjoying your meals? (For example: phones, watching TV, chatting, reading.)
  Ultimately, how and what we eat influences our digestion, our overall health, and our peace of mind. Cultivating well-being through mindful energy and tranquility is a core aim in all yogic practices.

Reflect

- What does your usual mealtime look like?
- Is there stress, rushing, or conflict involved?
- If so, what changes might you make to create a more mindful and peaceful eating experience?

Daily Lesson Plan #35: Ritual of Food

Intention/Objective
To share food in a peaceful joyous environment with an attitude of gratitude.
Teaching Resource Material
Sample Blessing for a Meal Handout
Review/Introduction
<ul><li>Discuss their experience of eating since the raisin exercise. What's changed, if anything?</li><li>Today we'll be sharing food together and experimenting with the idea of giving thanks before we dive into our meal.</li></ul>
Lesson
Centering:<ul><li>Wake up the digestive fire (Agni) with two minutes of seated jellyfish, side stretches and twisting.</li><li>The Boat/Navasana three times</li><li>Scale Asana/Lolasana (suspension bridge in Elementary Yoga Posters)</li><li>Side Plank/Vasisthasana</li><li>Revolved Head to Knee Asana/Janu Sirsasana</li><li>Partner Tree: Facing the same direction, slide your inside arm around your partner and hold onto their waist or shoulder. Ground through your foot/pada that's on the mat, bend your outer knee and tuck your outside foot into your inner thigh. After five or so breaths, switch sides.</li></ul>**Body of Class:**<ul><li>Turn off phones, no photos, no social media, no distractions.</li><li>Have various students read a few blessings from the handout or share any personal favorites.</li><li>Allow students to describe the dishes they prepared and other cultural eating rituals they have.</li><li>*This meal could also be shared in silence.</li></ul>**Closing:**<ul><li>Clean-up as a group activity with music.</li></ul>
Reflection/Conclusion
<ul><li>Did your food taste any different with a few moments of gratitude beforehand?</li><li>How did the experience of eating together differ from your usual eating habit?</li><li>What was it like eating food that your peers had created or curated themselves?</li></ul>
OMwork
Record any insights you've gained about food and list one enhancement to your diet that you can make that is both cost effective and nutritious. Add these items to your wellness portfolio.

You don't have to be religious—or wait for Thanksgiving—to appreciate the food in front of you. Taking a moment to say a blessing before eating is just a simple, intentional way to pause and recognize the gift of nourishment. It helps shift your focus from rushing to eating to really being present and thankful.

Here's something worth thinking about: around **830 million people** go to bed hungry every night, and every day **25,000 people**, including **10,000 children**, die from hunger. That makes every meal we get something truly worth appreciating.

Even something as easy as silently giving thanks or holding your bowl for a moment with gratitude can turn eating into a mindful, meaningful moment.

Here are a few playful options for blessing a meal:

An Attitude of Gratitude

Those who dine on hot dogs and pop,
With grins so wide they just can't stop,
Will likely thrive more than the brood
That sulks through every bite of "health" food.
   (Although this isn't entirely true because the quality of our food matters, it's a good argument for a joyful, grateful attitude when eating).

A Plea for Calorie Free

We give our thanks for this fine spread,
And humbly ask, as grace is said,
That heaven works its sweet concert—
To cleanse the calories from dessert.

A Blessing for a Bad Cook

   Bless this meal, whatever it is—
   I tried my best (no promises!).
   There's love in there… and maybe spice?
   Just take a bite and roll the dice.
   Send us grace, we might need that—
   I cooked with heart, but skills fell flat.
   So bless this food and all who munch,
   And please don't judge me *too* hard at lunch!

To the Delivery Person

   Big thanks for this awesome bite,
   Hot and fresh — it feels just right!
   Shoutout to the driver, brave and cool,
   For bringing the goods and making us drool!

A Blessing of Good Wishes

May the sun's soft light fall upon you,
And may tender love surround you.
May the light within your spirit glow,
And guide you where you need to go.

Daily Lesson Plan #36: Anatomy of Asanas

Intention/Objective
Students will gain familiarity with the anatomical terms for bones and muscles.
Review/Introduction
This class will focus on the physical anatomy of the human body, mainly comprehension of the major muscles and bones through individual movement and partner activities.
Lesson

Centering:
• Sun Salutation A and B three times, holding each asana to notice which muscle is contracting/shortening and which muscle is extending/lengthening.
Body of Class:
• Balancing Game
   ○ Find a body shape that bears weight on the hands (carpals) and feet (tarsals)
   ○ Find a body shape that bears weight on one hand and one foot
   ○ Find a body shape that bears weight on just the feet
   ○ Find a body shape that bears weight on your seat (ischial tuberosities/sits bones)
   ○ Find a shape that bears weight on body parts that don't include the feet or the hands.
   ○ Find a body shape that bears weight on soft tissue alone… (the Bow/Dhanurasana on the belly)
• In partners:
   ○ Create a partner asana that bears weight on three body parts collectively. Identify the anatomical terms of these body parts.
   ○ Create a partner asana that bears weight on two body parts. Identify the anatomical terms of these body parts.
   ○ Create a partner asana that bears weight on one body part. Identify the anatomical term of this body part.
• In groups of 3 or 4:
   ○ Create a group asana that has four body parts in contact with the floor.
   ○ Create a group asana that has three body parts in contact with the floor.
   ○ Create a group asana that has two body parts in contact with the floor.
   ○ Create a group asana that has as little contact with the floor as possible.
• Student-led Hokey Pokey Song- use proper anatomy terms for the body parts 'put in' to the centre.
Closing:
• Settle into a relaxing body form of your choosing and notice what body parts make contact with your mat. Let them sink into the earth and become heavy. Notice if you feel more connected to your body as your understanding of anatomy deepens.
• Quiet your mind and rest your attention on your breath.

Reflection/Conclusion
"If we can see each other as skeletons, We peel away the layers of what society deems as supreme. The mind's eye will not see differences, no comparisons will be made, Corralling fear and making space to love all equally, without judgement." ~ Colette Sampson MacLean
OMwork
• Review the Musculo-skeletal system and reflect on the importance of this knowledge for deepening your yoga practice. • The more you use anatomical terms, the more familiar they become, so start practicing! • Complete the Anatomy of an Asana Assignment

Daily Lesson Plan #36:
Anatomy of Asanas

OMwork Material
• Anatomy: The Skeletal and Muscular Systems Handout • Anatomy of an Asana Assignment Handout • Anatomy of an Asana Assignment Rubric

Anatomy: The Skeletal and Muscular Systems

As you deepen your Yoga practice, it's natural to become curious about the intricate details of our bodies—how they move and work together as a whole. To appreciate this complexity, consider that the human body is made up of approximately 100 trillion cells.

A strong foundation for understanding movement comes from exploring the locomotor system, which primarily consists of the **muscles** and **bones**.

Note: In yoga, you are learning three languages simultaneously:
- English terms related to the practice
- Sanskrit names for yoga postures (asanas)
- Anatomical terminology to describe the body

Therefore, be patient with yourself and stay curious about this learning process.

The Skeletal System

The skeletal system provides the body's structure and enables movement. Imagine what we would be without bones—a shapeless mass of soft tissue.
- The adult human body contains **206 bones**.
- The skeletal system is divided into two main parts:
    - **Axial skeleton**: This includes the central axis of the body—the skull, spinal column, and rib cage.
    - **Appendicular skeleton**: This includes the limbs—the arms and legs.

Bones grow stronger through **stress** or **weight-bearing activities**, which is why daily physical exercise is essential for maintaining healthy bones.

Bone Shapes

Bones come in three general shapes:
1. **Long bones** (e.g., femur) and **short bones** (e.g., carpals in the wrist)
2. **Flat bones** (e.g., cranial bones of the skull)
3. **Irregular bones** (e.g., vertebrae in the spine)

There are bones and muscles on the **anterior/front** and **posterior/back** plane of the body.

The 23 main bones are:
1. Cranium/skull
2. Mandible/jaw
3. Clavicle/collarbone
4. Scapula/shoulder blade
5. Humerus/upper arm
6. Radius/forearm, thumb side
7. Ulna/forearm, elbow side
8. Carpals/8 wrist bones

9. Metacarpals/hand bones
10. Phalanges/fingers
11. Sternum/Breastbone
12. Costae/Ribs
13. Ilium/hip bones
14. Sacrum/tailbone plate
15. Pubis/front pubic bone
16. Ischium/sits bones
17. Femur/thigh bones
18. Patella/kneecaps
19. Tibia/inner shin
20. Fibula/outer shin
21. Tarsals/ankle bones
22. Metatarsals/foot bones
23. Phalanges/toes

Bony prominences (heads of bones that stick out) serve as useful landmarks when learning about the skeletal system.

In pairs, explore the following prominences and identify the names of the bones you contact:
- Head of the humerus
- Spine of the scapula
- Iliac crest
- Greater Trochanter
- Medial and lateral Condyles of the knee
- Medial and lateral Malleoli: ankle bones

The **Muscular System**, with its 600 muscles, gives mobility to our bone structure so we can scratch an itch or leap to avoid oncoming traffic. Our muscular system also helps us to maintain **proper posture** and muscular movement creates **heat in the body**.

Three types of muscles:
1. Smooth/involuntary muscles (found in internal organs)
2. Cardiac/heart muscles
3. Skeletal/voluntary muscles (main muscles used during movement)

Movements of the body that you can do together as a class:
- Flexion and extension
- Abduction and Adduction
- Internal and External rotation
- Supination and Pronation

7 Major Anterior Muscles:
1. Deltoids/shoulder muscles
2. Pectorals/chest muscles
3. Biceps/upper arm muscles
4. Abdominals/core muscles
5. Iliopsoas/hip flexor muscles
6. Quadriceps/upper leg muscles

7 Major Posterior Muscles:

1. Trapezius/upper/mid back muscles
2. Rhomboids/mid back muscles
3. Latissimus Dorsi/outer back muscles
4. Triceps/back arm muscles
5. Gluteal/buttock muscles
6. Hamstrings/posterior upper leg muscles
7. Gastrocnemius/calf muscles

Additional muscle group:
- Pubococcygeal/pelvic floor muscles, which engage during Mula Bandha

Anatomy of an Asana Assignment

Curriculum Outcomes

By completing this assignment, students will:
- Demonstrate foundational standing, balance, seated, and supine postures with proper alignment.
- Show understanding of anatomy and physiology as it relates to the intentional integration of breath, posture, and movement in yoga practice.
- Identify asanas that align with their personal health goals and design a yoga practice for use outside of class.

Assignment Overview

For this project, you will create a poster that displays a yoga asana in perfect alignment, highlighting the skeletal bones involved.

Steps to Complete the Assignment

1. **Select an Asana:** Choose one posture from the 50 foundational asanas.
2. **Demonstrate Proper Alignment:** Ensure you can perform the asana correctly with proper alignment.
3. **Title Your Poster:** Include both the English and Sanskrit names of your chosen asana.
4. **Visual Representation:** Include a clear photo of yourself in the posture, a hand-drawn illustration, or a sourced image on your poster.
5. **Label Anatomy:** Identify and label the 23 main bones and 15 major muscles involved in the posture.
6. **Alignment Tips:** Write three detailed alignment tips for the asana. Cite all sources used for this information on the back of your poster (see citation guidelines below).
7. **Health Benefits:** List three health benefits associated with the asana. Research carefully and cite your sources.
8. **Design:** Be creative! Use colored paper, drawings, or graphics to make your poster visually appealing and unique. Use font and sizes of text that are easy to read and summarize the content clearly.

Citation Guidelines

When citing your sources, include the following information:
- Author
- Title of the article (including the website name)
- Date of publication
- Name of the website
- Full web address (URL)

Anatomy of an Asana Rubric

Requirement	0 points	1 point	2 points	3 points	4 points
Does photo demonstrate proper alignment?	Somewhat	Mostly	Completely		
Were the English and Sanskrit names included?	Neither English or Sanskrit	Either English or Sanskrit	Both English and Sanskrit		
Were tips included for proper alignment?	No tips	1 tip	2 tips	3 tips	
Were health benefits included?	No benefits	1 benefit	2 benefits	3 benefits	
How many bones and muscles were correctly labelled?	Less than 10	10 to 15	15 to all bones and muscles	All 23 bones and 15 muscles	
Does the poster display Photo arrangement Text size/font Clear, concise info Colourfulness	No design elements	1 design element	2 design elements	3 design elements	All design elements

Anatomy of an Asana Assessment

PROJECT DUE DATE STUDENT'S NAME	PHOTOS	ASANA NAMES	ALIGNMENT TIPS	HEALTH BENEFITS	BONES AND MUSCLES LABELS	DESIGN ELEMENTS	TOTAL (17)
1							
2							
3							
4							
5							
6							
7							
8							
9							
10							
11							
12							
13							
14							

Daily Lesson Plan #36:
Anatomy of Asanas

15								
16								
17								
18								
19								
20								
21								
22								
23								
24								

Daily Lesson Plan #37: Researching Systems

Intention/Objective
Students will gain understanding of the muscular, skeletal, respiratory, endocrine, urinary, integumentary (skin), cardiovascular, immune, digestive, reproductive and nervous systems of the body.
Teaching Resource Material
Systems of the Body Handout
Review/Introduction
<ul><li>In groups of three or four, students will be assigned a system of the body to research and prepare a five-minute presentation for the next class.</li><li>We will be researching a specific system of the body by answering the questions below. Be thoughtful about your sources and cite your references.</li></ul>
Lesson
The five questions to answer through your research are: 1. What is the system's function and role within the body? 2. Where is it located within the body? 3. What are the conditions or illnesses that can arise when this system is not functioning properly? 4. How is this system influenced by the practice of yoga and mindfulness? 5. What are three asanas that balance this system? What additional interesting facts have you learned through your research?
Reflection/Conclusion
After the students finish their research, come together for a group Om and then disperse.
OMwork
Preparations for the presentation.
OMwork Material
<ul><li>Systems of the Body Handout</li><li>Assessment for Systems Presentation</li></ul>

Systems of the Body

The Systems of the Body

- Muscular
- Skeletal
- Respiratory
- Cardiovascular
- Nervous
- Endocrine
- Immune / Lymphatic
- Excretory / Urinary
- Digestive
- Reproductive

- Integumentary (Skin)

Peer-Assessment for Systems Presentation

Was the system sufficiently researched, was the presentation informative? Give examples.
Did it relate to the practice of Yoga? Give examples.
What improvements could be made to make the presentation more effective/interesting?
What specific details of the presentation did you appreciate?

Daily Lesson Plan #38: Presentations

Intention/Objective
Students will present their findings on their assigned system of the body.:
Teaching Resource Material
Assessment for Systems Presentation
Review/Introduction
Two classes may be required to complete all presentations and leave time for questions at the end. Have the visual arts department video record each presentation for self-assessment afterward.
Lesson
Centering: Fun Facts about the human body: • The longest bone in the body is…the femur. • The smallest bone in the body is…the stirrup in the inner ear. • One quarter of all your bones live in…your feet. • The human head weighs…7-12lbs. • The strongest muscle in your body is…the tongue. • The body part that continues to grow throughout life is…your nose. • When you sneeze, the bodily functions that stop operating are…all of them, (even the heart) • A one-minute kiss burns…(30)…calories. **Body of Class:** Presentation of Systems of the Body – hand out 11 Peer-Assessments for each system and group.
Reflection/Conclusion
• **Legs up the wall/Viparita Karani** or **Relaxation/Savasana** with fall out breaths, let your body relax and take a moment to acknowledge your achievement today. • How will this information on your body's systems change the way you treat your body? • Can you see why yogis call their bodies a temple? Its construction is magnificent.
OMwork
• Choose three yoga asanas, one for warm up, one for the body of a class and one for cool down. Come to class tomorrow ready to share your asanas with a partner. • Reflect on The Voice of the Ego vs The Voice of the Self and identify in your journal what The Voice of the Ego sounds like and what The Voice of the Self says.
Omwork Material
Read Article: The Voice of the Ego versus the Self

The Ego versus the Self

The habit of constantly trying to please others often leads us to sacrifice our own needs, hoping that in return, others will fulfill those needs for us. This way of living is exhausting because it makes us dependent on external approval and validation. This is what it means to live an externally referenced life—where our sense of worth hinges on the opinions of others or societal expectations. Such a lifestyle pushes us into consumerism, convincing us that acquiring certain things or status will earn us love and acceptance.

However, the world is always changing, demanding that we continually consume, compete, and prove ourselves. This is the domain of the ego, which thrives on creating division through comparison and criticism. The ego convinces us that our value depends on our wealth, intelligence, appearance, social circle, and what others think of us.

The problem with living this way is that these measures are fleeting and largely beyond our control, leaving us constantly chasing a sense of belonging. When our sense of self is tied to external validation, we become vulnerable to others' opinions and labels, which are unpredictable and uncontrollable.

Consider how you might sacrifice your own needs to please others under peer pressure—in areas like social media, sexuality, substance use, body image, excessive training, or competition.

In yoga, this kind of living is called *dukkha*—a state of suffering or dissatisfaction—because we rely on others to bring us happiness.

Living from within, or being internally referenced, is quite different. When we turn inward and connect with the inherent goodness within ourselves, listening to our true needs and desires, we find genuine fulfillment and ease in our own skin.

By honoring our authentic needs and living in harmony with our highest values, we align with the voice of the self. Connected to our deepest essence, we tap into the universal current of love that flows through everything.

In yoga, this state is known as *sukha*—happiness, ease, or bliss—a condition we cultivate by choice. When we root ourselves in our inner power, the judgments of others lose their hold, allowing us to create a life filled with purpose, meaning, and peace.

How can you shift from dukkha/suffering to Sukha/happiness by altering your mindset?

Daily Lesson Plan #39:
Internal/SELF-Referenced Living

Intention/Objective
In this class, we'll be exploring the difference between living an internally referenced life (which tends to bring happiness or sukha) versus an externally referenced life (which undoubtedly brings discontent or dukkha).
Teaching Resource Material
Article: The voice of the ego versus the voice of the self.
Review/Introduction
<ul><li>Discuss the Omwork Article: The voice of the ego vs the voice of the self.</li><li>In this class, we'll be exploring the difference between living an internally referenced life (which tends to bring happiness or sukha) versus an externally referenced life (which undoubtedly brings discontent or dukkha).</li><li>It must be noted that while Ayurveda, the ancient sister science to yoga, claims that internally referenced living is important for our ultimate happiness, it's also essential to be open to feedback from our peers and people who care about us. We must learn to follow our own compass, (which is difficult today with so many external influences shaping our desires), while remaining curious about the impact of our behaviour on others.</li></ul>
Lesson
In partners, lead your partner through the three postures you chose for warm up, peak and cool down. Remember to hold asanas for 5-7 breaths. **20-minute Practice Teaching Class**<ul><li>This class will be led by the instructor today and can be used by the students to practice teach the next day.</li><li>Let's focus on the feeling of the asanas, flowing with the breath and healing injuries (internally referenced) instead of trying to perform to a certain standard, look good or gain positive attention (externally referenced).</li></ul>**Warm up:**<ul><li>Sun Breath</li><li>Sun Salutation A 1x</li><li>Sun Salutation B 1x</li></ul>**Standing Asanas:**<ul><li>Padangusthasana (Standing Forward Fold)</li><li>Virabhadrasana 2 (Warrior 2)</li><li>Parsvakonasana (Extended Side Angle)</li></ul>**Standing Balance Asana:**<ul><li>Vrksasana (Tree)</li></ul>**Seated Asanas:**<ul><li>Paschimottanasana (Seated Forward Bend)</li><li>Baddha Konasana (Bound Angle)</li></ul>**Closing Asanas:**<ul><li>Supta Parivartanasana (Supine Twist)</li><li>Savasana (Corpse)</li></ul>

Daily Lesson Plan #39:
Internal/SELF-Referenced Living

Reflection/Conclusion
"Like a solid rock is not shaken by the wind, so the wise are not moved by praise or blame." Buddha
OMwork
<ul><li>Next class, agree to try a no-brand name clothing class.</li><li>The Treasure Within story and the questions to go with the story.</li><li>Write a half page reflection on The Treasure Within story and the subsequent questions, outlining how it relates to your life.</li></ul>
OMwork Materials
Additional work on this topic, video: 'The Story of Stuff' 'The Treasure Within' story and 'Questions to go with Treasure Story'

The Treasure Within

There once was a man who longed to discover great treasures. He believed, deep in his soul, that riches awaited him somewhere in the world. So, with hopeful eyes and a restless heart, he set off on a journey to find his fortune.

He chased every lead, roaming far and wide—through bustling cities, across frigid mountain peaks, beneath the scorching desert sun. He dug through sands, wandered dense green forests, and cast his nets into the vast and open seas.

Years passed. The search was long, costly, and exhausting. Eventually, worn down and weary, with an empty wallet and a heavy heart, the man returned home. He had found no treasure—at least, not the kind he expected.

Time slipped by quietly as he settled back into his simple life. Then, one day, there was a knock at the door. An old friend had come to visit after many years apart.

While the dog slept soundly at their feet and the fireplace crackled, they sat together in the living room, rehashing old memories. As they talked, the friend's eyes drifted to the side table, where a rough stone held down a stack of papers.

"Where did you find that?" the friend asked, pointing.

"Oh, that old thing?" the man said casually. "I found it in the garden. It had a good weight to it, so I brought it in to use as a paperweight."

The friend leaned forward, with her eyes wide. "Do you know what that is?"

The man shrugged. "Just a rock from the backyard."

"No, my friend," the guest said with awe. "That's a raw diamond—likely worth millions."

The man had spent his life searching the world for treasure, never realizing it had been in his own backyard all along.

The truth is, we all carry treasures within us. Our worth isn't something we need to chase—it already lives inside us.

The jewel within you is waiting to be seen, valued, and discovered.

"Yoga does not just change the way we see things, it transforms the person who sees." — B.K.S. Iyengar

Questions to go with Treasure Story

1. What do you seek outside of yourself that you believe is not found within?
2. We all have treasures within, which are revealed through our natural talents. What are your top three gifts?

Daily Lesson Plan #39:
Internal/SELF-Referenced Living

3. Ask your friends and family members what they think are your top three gifts and record your results.

Realize that these are your superpowers that are totally unique to you, which may help to clarify your career path and contribute positively to the world.

Daily Lesson Plan #40: Yoga Flow Design

Intention/Objective
This class will be dedicated to creating a 20-minute yoga class, in partners.
Teaching Resource Material
<ul><li>Yoga Class Outline Handout</li><li>Practice Teaching Guideline Handout</li></ul>
Review/Introduction
Centering:<ul><li>Take a moment to tune in to the wisdom of your breathing, letting your body relax and your mind quiet down. Let go of any distractions so you can be fully present here. Reflect on the lesson last day and the challenge of being self-referenced in an object-referenced world.</li><li>Did you remember to wear no brand-named clothing?</li><li>Discuss *The Treasure Within* and how it applies to your life.</li><li>This class will be spent with a partner, designing your own 20-minute yoga class that consists of a warm-up and eight asanas. You can use the last class as a guide, as it included a few namaskar, followed by eight asanas. Clarify the asana categories they must include, shown in the yoga class framework.</li><li>Invite the students to create a playlist of various genres to suit the different phases of a class. For example, warm-up music would be slow and melodic and then build to more upbeat music for the stronger asanas and finally flow into reflective music for the closing part of the class.</li></ul>
Lesson
Centering:<ul><li>Student-led Namaskars in partners.</li></ul>**Body of Class:**<ul><li>As a class, agree to the parameters of this assignment:<ul><li>Cooperation between partners, in choosing asanas and music</li><li>Choose eight asanas from the 50 Foundational Asanas, within your ability to demonstrate</li><li>Choose music that aligns with the principles of yoga (no violent or oppressive lyrics)</li><li>Length of class is 20 minutes, so divide teaching time evenly with your partner</li><li>Each asana is held for five to seven breaths, closing postures can be held longer</li><li>Instruct the right side first, then the left side</li><li>Include the transitions between asanas in your planning</li></ul></li><li>Assessment will be based on asanas chosen, participation and leadership</li></ul>**Closing:** Savasana or a closing asana of your choice. Reflection: may this work help to create a world where people feel safe and secure with a deep sense of belonging to this human community.
Reflection/Conclusion
<ul><li>Sitting appreciations: With hands in Namaste, share one thing you appreciate about your partner during this process.</li><li>Notice how it felt to incorporate creativity, partner work and independence into your practice.</li></ul>

Daily Lesson Plan #40:
Yoga Flow Design

• What did you discover about sequencing asanas? What worked, what didn't?
OMwork
Prepare to present your yoga class next class.
OMwork Material
Yoga Class Outline Handout Practice Teaching Guideline Handout

Yoga Class Outline Handout: 20-minute Peer-Led Practice Teaching Class

Date:
Teachers:
Props:
Warm up: 2 Namaskaras
Standing Asanas: 3 asanas

Daily Lesson Plan #40: Yoga Flow Design

Standing Balance Asana: 1 asana

Seated Asanas: 2 asanas

Closing Asanas: 2 asanas, 1 being Savasana

Reflection/Conclusion
Reflect on your teaching and answer the following questions:
What parts went well?
What will you do differently next time you lead?
When receiving, did you support your peers with kindness and attention?

OMwork Material

Daily Lesson Plan #40:
Yoga Flow Design

Practice Teaching Guideline

Curriculum Outcomes

- Apply effective breathing techniques in personal yoga practice.
- Identify asanas aligned with desired health benefits and develop a yoga sequence for use outside of class.
- Demonstrate understanding of the Eight Limbs of Ashtanga Yoga.
- Explore relaxation methods to observe thoughts, manage emotions and stress, and reflect on which techniques work best.
- Integrate the principles of yoga personally beyond class practice.

Assignment Overview

For your final evaluation in Yoga 11, you will design a personalized asana class and curate a complementary yoga playlist that reflects your experience in the course.
- **Music Selection:**
- Your playlist should embody your intention behind the practice while honoring **Ahimsa**—nonviolence, compassion, and kindness—not only towards yourself but also for others in the class.
- **Playlist:**
- Create a playlist lasting 20–45 minutes that you would be happy to return to for your personal practice in the future.

Playlist Requirements

Include musical pieces for the following phases of your class:
- Grounding/Centering with Breathwork
- Asana Practice (reflecting your class intention with gradual pacing: warm-up, main sequence, cool down)
- Relaxation/Savasana

Suggested Class Structure

- **Grounding/Centering:** Set your intention for the practice.
- **Breathwork/Breath Awareness:** Focus on mindful breathing techniques.
- **Warm-Up Asanas:** Examples include Child's Pose, Seated Twist, Mountain Pose, Namaskars.
- **Main Sequence Asanas:** Incorporate standing postures, standing balances, and perhaps arm balances.
- **Cool Down:** Examples include Supine Twist (Jathara Parivartanasana), Knees to Chest (Apanasana), Half Bridge (Setu Bandhasana).
- **Relaxation/Savasana:** Final resting posture for integration and peace.

Daily Lesson Plan #41: Yoga Class Presentations

Intention/Objective
Students will join with another set of partners and present the yoga class that they've designed and also participate in their peer-led yoga classes.   **Teaching Resource Material:**   Peer Assessment Handout
Review/Introduction
Review the parameters for the 20-minute peer-led yoga class.   If possible, disperse into quiet rooms or hallways so they can play their playlist while they flow.
Lesson
Yoga Class Presentations   First and foremost, as you lead your class, you are instructed to practice self-compassion, by giving yourself grace and treating yourself respectfully throughout this exercise. We're not seeking perfection, we're seeking progress.   Students have up to 20 minutes to present their class to their set of partners.   Classmates can offer constructive, mostly positive feedback after each presentation.   *Option to record or photograph their yoga teaching for self-assessment, teacher assessment and/or classroom decoration.   **Peer Assessment**   Did the presenters demonstrate proper alignment in their asanas?   Did they demonstrate the ethical yogic principles while leading the class?   What creative aspects did you notice and appreciate?   Was self-compassion evident throughout their teaching?   **Closing**   Self-compassion practice: Take a final moment to let your breath drop into your body and acknowledge your dedication to showing up and pushing your growing edge. Feel free to rest one or both hands on your heart space and think about three-character qualities that you appreciate about yourself in this moment. Be generous with yourself and record your answers.   Namaste or high five at least three people, congratulating them on their presentations.
Reflection/Conclusion
Let celebration be a regular part of your life, especially when you do something that pushes your comfort zone, like you did today (note that there are healthy ways of celebrating).
OMwork
Journal entry: Who would you be and what would you do if you stepped out of your own way?
Omwork Material
Chakra Handout

Peer Assessment Handout

Date:
Teachers:
Did the presenters demonstrate proper alignment in their asanas?
Did they demonstrate the ethical yogic principles while leading the class?
What creative aspects did you notice and appreciate?
Was self-compassion evident throughout their teaching?
What suggestions would you offer for their next teaching adventure?

Daily Lesson Plan #41:
Yoga Class Presentations

Chakra Handout

In the yoga tradition, *Chakra*s are described as wheels or vortexes of energy that correspond to nerve bundles and major organs in the body. When these so-called 'spinning disks' of energy are healthy, they are open and aligned, which affect our emotional and physical well-being.

There are seven main chakras that run along the spinal column, each with a corresponding name, color, sound, health focus and specific location.

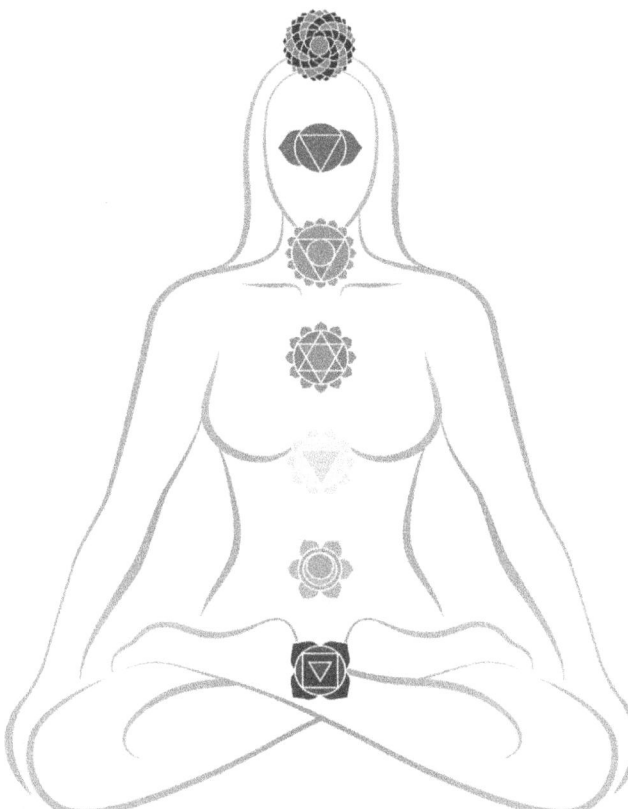

Seventh Chakra
Color: Cloud white or violet
Location: Crown of head / brain
Meaning: Unity awareness, peace and bliss

Sixth Chakra
Color: Deep purple/indigo
Location: Mid-brow / third eye
Meaning: Intuition, imagination, concentration

Fifth Chakra
Color: Sky blue
Location: Throat
Meaning: Communication and self-expression

Fourth Chakra
Color: Grassy green
Location: Heart center
Meaning: Emotion, love and connection

Third Chakra
Color: Golden yellow
Location: Upper abdomen
Meaning: Self-esteem and self-confidence

Second Chakra
Color: Bright orange
Location: Beneath the navel
Meaning: Self-worth and creativity

Root Chakra
Color: Earthy red
Location: Base of spine/tailbone
Meaning: Personal identity, security and grounding

Daily Lesson Plan #42: Student Teaching

Intention/Objective
Students will apply their understanding of yoga and test their leadership by teaching younger children.
Teaching Resource Material
Review/Introduction
In new partners, students will prepare a 25–30-minute yoga class for children of younger grades, incorporating the chakras and their colors.
Lesson
<ul><li>With your partner, brainstorm things to consider when preparing to teach a class (time, environment, availability of props, participant ability, age etc).</li><li>Using the analogy of a mountain, every class contains a warm-up as you climb the mountain, then the body of the class occurs at the top with a peak posture, with a cool down phase as you hike down the mountain.</li><li>Warm-up usually includes a namaskar, the body includes standing and standing balance asanas, and the cool down includes seated or supine asanas.</li><li>Create an age-appropriate lesson, using asanas from the 50 Foundational Asanas and the Elementary posters, if available.</li><li>When designing your class, include the chakra(s) targeted for each asana, using the Chakra Handout as a reference.</li><li>Incorporate the chakra colors into your class.</li><li>Arrange for a date to do these student-led classes with local schools, once the lessons have been approved by the teacher.</li></ul>
Reflection/Conclusion
<ul><li>What did you like about preparing this class?</li><li>What did you enjoy about teaching Yoga to the younger grades?</li><li>What did you find challenging about teaching Yoga to younger kids?</li><li>Can you see yourself teaching Yoga one day?</li></ul>
OMwork
Make a list of qualities you believe an effective yoga instructor possesses.
OMwork Material
<ul><li>Asana Chart Handout</li><li>Practice Teaching Reflection</li></ul>

Asana Flow Chart

Asana Sequence Assignment Instructions

1. Visual Layout

- Create a stick figure drawing of each asana in its own box.
- Below each drawing, include:
  - **Name of the posture** (Sanskrit + English if possible)

- One **teaching point** for proper alignment
- **Chakra involved**

2. Select 10 Postures

   Your sequence must include:
   1. **1 Mindfulness Asana** (Centering)
   2. **1 Surya Namaskar or Classical Salutation** (Warm-up)
   3. **2 Standing Asanas**
   4. **1 Standing Balance Asana** (Peak)
   5. **2 Seated Asana**
   6. **1 Core Asana**
   7. **1 Supine Asana**
   8. **1 Savasana** (Closing)

3. Partner Work

   With your teaching partner:
   - Decide how you will **divide the teaching** (who teaches which postures or sections)
   - Explore how you will **incorporate the creativity of the chakras** (through cues, visualization, color, theme, etc.)
   - Plan how you will **explain and guide transitions** between postures
   - **Practice teach** your class together to ensure flow and timing

Daily Lesson Plan #42:
Student Teaching

Asana Chart

Name	
Mindfulness Asana Asana name: Teaching point: Chakra involved:	Surya Namaskar or Classical Salutation Asana name: Teaching point: Chakra involved:
Standing Asana 1 Asana name: Teaching point: Chakra involved:	Standing Asana 2 Asana name: Teaching point: Chakra involved:
Standing Balance Asana Asana name: Teaching point: Chakra involved:	Seated Asana 1 Asana name: Teaching point: Chakra involved:
Seated Asana 2 Asana name: Teaching point: Chakra involved:	Core Asana Asana name: Teaching point: Chakra involved:
Supine Asana Asana name: Teaching point: Chakra involved:	Savasana Asana name: Teaching point: Chakra involved:

Daily Lesson Plan #42:
Student Teaching

Practice Teaching Reflection

What did you like about preparing this class?

What did you enjoy about teaching Yoga to the younger grades?

What did you find challenging about teaching Yoga to younger kids?

Can you see yourself teaching Yoga one day? Why or why not?

Daily Lesson Plan #43:
Yoga Class in Nature

Intention/Objective
"Look deep into nature and you will understand everything better." ~ Albert Einstein
Review/Introduction
<ul><li>Take the class to a natural setting to practice yoga in the great outdoors. Encourage them to dress accordingly. If it's winter, find an indoor spot that has natural lighting, as close to nature as possible. If it's June, encourage them to stand on the earth in bare feet.</li><li>Discuss the five elements that inhabit every living creature, and that align with the chakras: Earth (first chakra), water (second chakra), Fire (third chakra), air (fourth chakra), space (fifth chakra).</li><li>Remain aware of these elements as you flow through your practice.</li></ul>
Lesson
Energizing Vinyasa Class **Centering:**<ul><li>Set an intention for your outdoor practice</li><li>Quote: "Nature does not hurry yet everything is accomplished." ~ Lao Tzu</li><li>Breath of Joy, taking in the healing properties of nature</li><li>Surya Namaskar A - as you sweep arms overhead, draw the shape of the sun, as you rise to standing, imagine growing upward like a tree on a mountain.</li><li>Surya Namaskar B - create space in your body and air in your lungs, breathing fresh oxygenated air (space and air elements).</li><li>Notice: If you're starting to sweat, this is the fire and water elements at work.</li></ul>**Body of Class:**<ul><li>Powerful/Utkatasana - what aspects of nature look like this? A lightning bolt?</li><li>Lunge/Anjaneyasana to Twisting Lunge or Revolved Side Angle/Parsvakonasana (grounding postures activate earth element)</li><li>Warrior 1, stepping forward into Eagle/Garudasana: how focused can you remain even in the strongest winds (air)? Can you root down (earth element)?</li><li>Seated Staff/Dandasana</li><li>Seated Forward Fold/Paschimottanasana - feel the calm, cool nature of this asana</li><li>Inverted Table/Bharmanasana - let the torso open to the energy of the sun</li><li>Head to Knee/Janu Sirsasana -feel your body close to the powerful energy of the earth.</li><li>Seated Twist/Ardha Matsyendrasana, with bottom leg extended or tucked (twists help to release gas from colon, air element:)</li><li>The Boat/Navasana - breathe deeply and create fire in your core.</li><li>The Crow/Bakasana - let your hands become your anchor, your foundation</li><li>Jump back from the Crow to Chaturanga Dandasana/Four Limbed Staff</li></ul>**Closing:**<ul><li>Bound Angle/Baddha Konasana - let the knees flap like the wings of a butterfly</li><li>Half Bridge/Setu Bandhasana - feel the strength of the backside support the lengthening of the front side</li><li>Supine Twist/Jathara Parivartanasana - twist like the twisted root of a tree</li><li>Knee to Chest, one leg at a time, and then both knees/Apanasana - tuck into a ball like an acorn or a berry</li><li>Relaxation/Savasana—Open your senses to the sights, sounds, scents and textures of nature, it is buzzing with life and energy.</li><li>Read *Reconnecting with Nature* Poem below</li></ul>

Reflection/Conclusion
• Reflect on how you feel amidst the natural world (it typically calms and regulates us). • Reflect on the importance of connecting to nature (improves our health, improves our connection to nature, making us more inclined to protect it). • Brainstorm things we can do, or steps we can take to live with a deeper sense of connection to the natural world (buy house plants, walk daily, practice outside, spend social time in the outdoors etc)
OMwork
• Take time daily to explore the natural world, by gazing up into the starry night sky, soaking in a sunset by the ocean, lying on your back and smelling the freshly cut grass, practicing mindfulness outdoors and listen to the sound of birds and flowing water, smelling the fragrances of nature, noticing the shades and colors and feeling the different textures. • Record how you feel after our outdoor yoga class vs doing yoga indoors.
OMwork Material
Reconnecting with Nature poem

Reconnecting with Nature

We've been led to believe that to truly connect with nature,
We need the right gear, the right brands and the perfect setting.
But the truth is—we don't need high-tech tools or stunning landscapes.
We don't have to conquer mountain peaks or dive into unknown waters,
Pretending to love the risk, the chase or even the solitude.

When we arrive at our destination, we might still feel empty—
Still pulled by the reflex to scroll,
Because no matter where we go, we bring ourselves along—
And the invisible burdens we carry within.

But nature doesn't ask for anything from us.
She has no test to pass, no standard to meet—
No beauty requirements or levels of fitness to achieve.
To connect, all we must do is step outside,
Sit quietly and listen with an open heart.

She speaks in birdsong, in breezes, in the gentle rush of water.
Connection happens by lying back on a bed of grass,
Letting our tension melt into the earth's soft cradle.
It's remembering that we are part of her—
A single wave in her ocean, a single leaf on her tree.

This is the belonging we long for.
All she asks is that we show up, just as we are—
To witness her colors, breathe in her scents,
And honor her gifts with care and reverence.

Daily Lesson Plan #44:
Yin Yoga for Self-love

Teaching Resource Materials
• Sample Movement Class from Mindfulness in Schools Manual • Two blocks and a band for each student.
Introduction
Yin yoga, unlike our typical vinyasa or yang-style practices, has a very different flavour and feel. Instead of holding each posture for 5–8 breaths, yin asanas are held for **3–5 minutes**, allowing the body to soften and release more deeply. Most asanas are practiced close to the ground, encouraging relaxation in joints that often carry deep-seated tension—particularly the hips and spine. **The defining elements of a yin yoga class include:** • Extended time spent in each asana • A slowing and deepening of the breath • Stillness in the body (as much as possible) • Mindful, gradual transitions between postures • The supportive use of props to help release tension
Lesson

Hero/Virasana with hands joined at heart center
Opening affirmations and reflections:
• I realize that when I open my heart to Love, life surprises me with goodness.
• **Fan the heart fire:**
   o Starting in Anjali mudra, inhale hands apart, exhale palms together for five to ten cycles. Add affirmation: "Breathing in I honor my heart, breathing out I fill it with love."
   o Continue this movement, as the teacher reads the following dialogue: Now is the time to practice loving yourself. To truly love another, you must first be able to offer love to yourself. Loving others means embracing them exactly as they are—and self-love asks the same of you.
   o Let this be a space where you meet yourself just as you are, with kindness and acceptance. Appreciate the precious, one-of-a-kind being that you are.
• **Hero/Virasana:**
   o Interlock fingers with palms in your lap facing upward, inhale lift your hands up your midline turning palms open to gradually press overhead. Maintaining the interlock, exhale press palms out in front as you lower the hands. Take five to ten gentle breaths here.
• **Butterfly (Cobbler's asana):**
   o Come home to your body and gently notice how you're holding it—how you're breathing. In our busy lives, we often ignore the body's needs, forcing it to meet the mind's demands. We push too hard or not enough. We overeat, under-eat, numb discomfort with substances or distractions, and sacrifice rest for productivity.
   o We disconnect from parts of the body that hold pain or difficult memories. We override its messages with caffeine, sugar, medication, or alcohol—anything to avoid listening. In a culture that profits from body dissatisfaction, we're taught to criticize rather than care, to strive for impossible standards instead of honoring what we have.

Daily Lesson Plan #44: Yin Yoga for Self-love

- o This rejection takes a toll—not just mentally, but energetically. Dis-eased thinking can manifest as dis-ease in the body. But we can begin to shift this. The first step is simple, yet powerful: gratitude.
- o Be thankful for the body you have—not the one you wish you had, or think you should have—but this body, here and now. The one that breathes for you, carries you, and speaks to you, even when you haven't been listening. Begin again, with love.
- **Supine Cobbler's:**
  - o Your body is extraordinary—a marvel of natural engineering. It instantly defends against invading viruses and bacteria, skillfully digests food, and releases precisely the right hormones in just the right amounts—all happening simultaneously. Considering the millions of potential illnesses we could face; it's truly a miracle how beautifully our bodies keep us functioning every single moment.
- **Sphinx:**
  - o Breathe deeply into your belly and your heart, inviting self-acceptance, compassion, and love. Imagine that your body needs no changes to be worthy of love—that you can fully accept and cherish it just as it is, in all its unique beauty, right here, right now.
- **Child's:**
  - o As we release physical layers of tension, we begin to uncover the truth of who we are and what we're made of. Going deeper in an asana isn't about pushing to our limit—it's about softening into the posture, deepening our capacity for love, and expanding our understanding of ourselves.
- **Dragon:**
  - o Dialogue for the first side:
  - o Nothing truly worthwhile ever arises from criticism, judgment, or scrutiny. We don't awaken our inner light through force or harshness—in fact, addictive and obsessive behaviors often grow stronger in their presence. As yogis, we nurture our bodies with compassion, tenderness, and love.
  - o Dialogue for the second side:
  - o If you're yearning to feel okay just as you are, you've come to the right place—because that comfort already lives within you. This journey isn't about adding anything new; it's about letting go—releasing negativity and everything that no longer serves you.
  - o As the false layers fall away, what remains is your true, brilliant self. Our work isn't to change or become someone else, but simply to allow ourselves to be exactly who we are.
- **Twisted Dragon:**
  - o First side:
  - o I can only truly connect with another when I first become fully present with myself.
  - o Second side:
  - o I can only truly love another by first filling my own heart with love.
  - o When I open my heart to Love, I am embraced by delight and peace.
- **Swan (Pigeon):**
  - o With crossed wings to open the back door of the heart. Let go of the pain from the past so you can enjoy the love that is here for you today.
  - o On the other side, cross arms the other way as well.
  - o If self-love feels difficult, imagine extending love to someone you cherish deeply. Then gently turn that love inward.
  - o Our work on the mat often brings our tender places to the surface, so we can meet them with healing and care. You are already whole. Sometimes, all that's needed is a shift in how you relate to yourself.
  - o Throughout this practice, tune into your inner dialogue. When a harsh thought or comparison arises, simply observe it—and then question its truth.
  - o Over time, as your commitment to self-love deepens, your inner voice will grow softer, more compassionate. And one day, you'll recognize the truth: you're already enough, just as you are.

- **Caterpillar (Seated Forward Bend):**
    - You are invited to say goodbye to feeling bad about your body and appearance. Today is your chance to stop colluding with a culture that profits from your pain by convincing you that you're not enough. It's time to say goodbye to your inner critic—the voice that keeps you striving endlessly and never lets you rest in peace.
    - Your inner critic may have meant well, but the true path to love is through radical self-acceptance. It's called radical because it goes against the norm. We often misunderstand self-acceptance as apathy or laziness, but in truth, radical self-acceptance means being gentle, forgiving, and generous with yourself.
    - The next time you see your reflection, notice the story you tell yourself: too tall, too petite, too soft, too plain, too dark, too curvy, too average. Just listen to these thoughts as if you're standing at the edge of a pool—without jumping in.
    - When you look in the mirror again, simply see your face, your body, your temple. By choosing not to dive into the pool of self-criticism, you begin to see the real you—the one who glows with a light completely unique to you.
    - This is the first step in healing your relationship with your body and transforming how you show up in the world.
- **Pentacle (Savasana):**
    - Let's make a promise to ourselves—to be kinder, gentler, more loving.
    - As this transformation unfolds within you, imagine the ripple it creates—touching your family, your future children, your friends, your colleagues.
    - Your inner peace becomes a gift they receive, quietly inspiring them to heal their own relationship with their bodies.
    - By nurturing ourselves, we become beacons of peace, helping to heal the world—one heart at a time.

Closing Affirmation:

I am deserving of the same love I freely give to others.

I open my heart to welcome goodness and love into my life.

I choose to embrace and celebrate who I am.

Daily Lesson Plan #45:
Girl on Fire Empowerment Class

Teaching Resource Material
Girl on Fire Empowerment Movement Class - Raising Resilience
Lesson
<ul><li>Child's/Balasana</li><li>Hero/Virasana with Neck Stretches</li><li>Mountain/Tadasana with Fall Out Breaths</li><li>Arm Vinyasa (inhale arms out and up, exhale down the center with palms together)</li><li>Ragdoll forward fold</li><li>Wide legged forward fold with scalp massage</li><li>Wide legged forward fold with side stretch, hands reach to one leg, then to the other</li><li>Wide legged squat with twist</li><li>Classical Namaskar</li><li>Warrior 3/Virabhadrasana 3</li><li>Tree/Vrksasana</li><li>Feature Posture: Gather and Ground Flow, like arm vinyasa only the palms turn down as the hands lower</li><li>Locust three times, eventually with fingers interlocked behind back</li><li>Prone Saddle — single leg quad stretch on belly or side.</li><li>Upward Facing dog</li><li>Tabletop with cat/cow flow</li><li>Cow Face/Gomukhasana in Hero or full version</li><li>Partner Posture: Seated Wide Angle Forward fold, joining feet and hands with your partner.</li><li>Relaxation/Savasana</li></ul>**Girl on Fire closing:**<ul><li>Invite them to repeat after you to acknowledge the three centers of Power, Love and Insight: Rise to sitting and bring palms together.</li><li>Lift hands so that thumbs touch the mid eye point and say, "Guided by insight".</li><li>Now draw hands to heart, one palm on heart center in the middle of the chest and the other palm resting on top of the first hand and say, "I listen to my heart's desire".</li><li>Now take the top hand and slide it down so it rests on the navel, with the first hand remaining on the heart and say, "And take positive action in the world."</li></ul>

Daily Lesson Plan #46:
Yoga for Autism Energizing Class

This class is designed to awaken prana—life force energy—throughout all systems of the body. Chronic stress often shows up as physical tension, and when certain areas remain tense for long periods, they become armored, rigid, and deprived at the cellular level.

Through movement and muscle lengthening, yoga reawakens these neglected spaces, restoring them with energy and blood flow. While all exercise supports health, yoga is especially powerful due to its intentional breathwork, which delivers oxygen-rich nourishment to the brain and body—serving as true brain food.

In alignment with this class's stress-relieving and energizing theme, we'll explore asanas that support emotional release, such as the Drum.

Note: When a specific breath count is not provided, hold each posture for 5–8 breaths.

Intention/Objective
Students will demonstrate an understanding of asanas that release stress and awaken their energy.
Teaching Resource Material
• Sample Class from Yoga for Autism Curriculum co-authored by Jenny Kierstead & Catherine Rahey • Introductory Preparatory Story You can begin each yoga class with the following preparatory story; **All about learning yoga** *I am going to a yoga class where I will learn how to do yoga.* *There will be a yoga teacher showing me how to do yoga.* *_____ is my yoga educator.* *In yoga class I will learn how to move my body in different ways.* *Each movement of my body is called a yoga asana or posture.* *There are many different body shapes in yoga.* *Each shape will help me in special ways.* *Yoga asanas can help me:* *relax when I'm feeling stressed* *focus better on what I need to do* *give me energy when I am tired* *help prepare me for sleep* *Learning new yoga shapes takes a lot of practice. Sometimes it will be hard work, sometimes it will be easy. That is okay.* *I may not be able to do each asana the way the teacher does on my first try. I will need to practice the asana so I can do it better. That is okay too.* *It is important that I listen to my teacher's instructions and watch him/her with my eyes to see how s/he does each asana.* *After I watch and listen I will try the asana with my teacher. My teacher may need to help me move my body into the right position. This means that s/he may need to touch me. That is okay. Then I can try to do it just like my teacher.* *Practicing yoga will be a lot of fun.* *I will try to listen to my teacher's instructions and do the asanas just like him/her.* *Yoga will help me to be more relaxed, focused and happy.*

Daily Lesson Plan #46:
Yoga for Autism Energizing Class

Introduction Discussion
Discuss the things in students' lives that drain their energy such as times of the day, certain subjects in school, screen usage, dehydration, sleep deprivation, negative emotions, etc. Inform students that we all have an energy budget for each day. This class is designed to fill their tank with energy. Invite your students to give their energy levels a rating, one being no energy (running on empty) and 10 being completely charged (a full tank). They may want to record their rating for reference at the end of class.
Lesson

- **Opening Asanas:**
  - Introduce modified Alternate Nostril Breathing, inhaling through the right nostril and exhaling through the left for an energizing effect.
  - Bee Breathing
- **Warm up Asanas:**
  - Neck stretches
  - Table
  - Drum, on knees and forearms and tap the mat like a drum
  - Downward Dog
- **Standing Asanas:**
  - Mountain
  - Seaweed/Standing Forward Fold with Lion's Breath on the way down
- **Standing balance:**
  - Dancer
- **Core Asana:**
  - The Boat
- **Back bending:**
  - Snake (cobra) for 10 breaths
  - Ice cream bowl (the bow)
  - Turtle (child's)
- **Hip Opening:**
  - LeapFrog (jumping malasana)
  - Butterfly (Bound Angle)
- **Closing Asanas:**
  - Twisted Twizzler/Supine twist/Ardha Matsyendrasana
  - Sleeping Sloth/Savasana
- **Conclusion:**
  - Feel the new positive energy traveling through your body and mind. Identify the level of energy in your body now, on a scale of one to 10. Celebrate any progress (increases in energy, decreases in tension).
- **Song (optional):**

  Five Little Yogis—to the tune of Five Green and Speckled Frogs

  Five little yogis
  Strike out a yoga pose
  Tree, cobra, downward dog
  They all take a deep full breath
  And feel relaxed and calm
  Then they salute with Namaste

  Five little yogis
  Sit on their yoga mats
  Tree, cobra, downward dog
  One jumps into the crow
  Where he/she feels free and strong

And they salute with Namaste
Thank your classmates for sharing your yoga experience with your Peaceful Happy Heart and Namaste.
OMwork
Energy assignment: Take inventory of your energy levels morning, noon and evening, using the scale from one-10. Can you identify what drains and boosts your energy throughout the day? Explore with yoga exercises, like deep breathing upon waking or balance asanas after lunch.

Daily Lesson Plan #47:
Yoga for Diverse Learners, Happy Feet Class

This class was inspired by observing that many students with physical limitations often have weakened or misaligned feet. These asanas are designed to bring awareness to this commonly neglected part of the body—an area we often ignore or even feel disconnected from.

By relieving tension and activating the feet, we help build a stronger, more stable foundation for the entire body. As mindfulness of the feet increases, students learn to root down with intention, engaging the stabilizing muscles of the feet and lower legs with greater precision and support.

Teaching Materials
• This is a sample class from the *Yoga for Diverse Learners Manual*.   • A band and a chair for each student.
Outline for Class
• Introduce the theme of footcare   • Personal hygiene   • Easy Asana/Sukhasana   • Mountain/Tadasana   • Classical Namaskara   • Hero/Virasana   • Powerful/Utkatasana   • Downward Dog/Adho Mukha Svanasana   • Yogic Squat/Malasana   • Squirrel Climbing Tree/Supta Padangusthasana   • Partner Seated Wide Legged Stretch/Diamond/Upavista Konasana   • Toe Game   • Foot/Pada Mandala
Lesson
• Introduce the topic and ask the students what they think of feet?   • Take this opportunity to speak about personal hygiene and how important it is to clean the body regularly, especially on yoga days when you'll be taking your socks off.   • In Sukhasana, interdigitate the toes by placing fingers between each toe crease, initially at the fingertips and gradually sliding the toes right up to the root of the fingers, the thickest area. Add a foot massage with the free hand.   • Mountain: Lift the toes wide and lower only the big toes together, now lower just the pinky toes, can you lift and spread the middle three toes? Slowly lower them all to your mat and relax. Do you have yogi toes now?   • Classical Namaskar: As you lunge back, keep the toes tucked under to feel the stretch through the arches. Notice how we stretch the soles of the feet when the toes are tucked, in lunge or downward dog, and then notice how we stretch the tops of the feet in the cobra or upward facing dog. Which direction do you find more difficult, toes pointed or tucked?   • Hero/Virasana with toes tucked under and then with toes pointed. Using a towel beneath the feet might be necessary when they point the toes and sit on the tops of the feet.   • Powerful Asana/Utkatasana with heels lifted, arms up in front, parallel to the floor. In this version, the torso is upright so the shoulders stack over the hips and the hips stack over the heels which are lifted, and the weight is bearing on the balls of the feet.

- Downward Dog and peddle the feet to feel the difference in the stretch from one foot to another.
- Yogic Squat/Malasana—from Mountain, inhale arms overhead and lower the hands to heart center. Squat deeply with torso inside of the knees, lowering the head toward the floor in front of the toes with hands cupping the heels.
- Squirrel Climbing Tree/Supine leg stretch: Lying on your back, lift the right leg and interlock the fingers behind the thigh or calf. Circle the foot in one direction and then the other. Do the same with the other leg.
- Partner Upavista Konasana/Diamond Pose: With feet wide, partner A's feet touching partner B's feet. Join hands or forearms and sit up tall, rolling onto the sitting bones (versus leaning back on the tailbone). Explore the stretch with your partner's support.
- Toe Strengthening Game: Using cylindrical pool toys that look like mini batons, or pens, give students three and challenge them to use their feet to pick them up.

Final Quote: "If the only prayer you said in your whole life was 'thank you,' that would be enough." ~ Meister Eckhart

Daily Lesson Plan #48:
Trauma-sensitive Movement Practice

Intention/Objective
Why we need to be trauma-sensitive today: • 90% of the population have been exposed to a traumatic event • Rates of abuse and oppression in marginalized populations persists • Nobody wants to re-traumatize someone unintentionally • Leading any kind of contemplative practice, can have unintended consequences for those who are living with trauma
Teaching Resource Material
• This is a sample class from *Trauma-sensitive Mindfulness Training* • Soft music, closed doors, warm blankets and a reminder of the Yoga Class Agreements
Review/Introduction
Four C's of a Trauma-sensitive Presence Attunement is the ability to sense others so that we can respond in a way that accurately captures how they are feeling. Attunement helps us to feel seen, heard and understood. When we feel this way, we feel safe, and safety is the goal for any trauma-sensitive led experience. 1. **Consistency** - routine fosters trust and safety 2. **Choice** - giving the practitioner the freedom to choose 3. **Compassion** - understanding leads to patience and space 4. **Connection** - to inner self, to coping self and then to others
Lesson

The following is a gentle trauma-sensitive somatic practice that supports students in returning to their body and breath, in a safe and gradual way.
• **Soft Belly Breathing:**
  o Soften your belly, perhaps resting a hand over your belly button. Start by breathing into the collarbones, then into the ribcage and over time, you can let the breath drop into the belly.
• **Shaking:**
  o Stand comfortably and begin bouncing in the knees, shaking the hands, arms, shoulders and head.
• **Hands to Heart:**
  o Resting palms together in front of the heart, take a few breaths and let the hands follow the breath, in your own way.
• **Cloud Hands:**
  o Sweep one hand across in front of the chest as the lower hand sweeps across in front of the abdomen. On the next breath, switch hand placement.
• **Figure 8:**
  o Imagine your sit bones have pencils attached and you want to draw a figure 8 on the floor beneath you. start moving the hips front to back, then switch.
• **Sitting Sprint:**
  o Start slowly, in a stationary walk, then increase the pace by sprinting as fast as you can. After a few strong deep breaths at a sprint, slow the pace again until you're sitting in stillness.

- **Crane:**
  - Like the majestic bird with the grand wingspan, flap your wings gently and lift onto one foot as you pulse the arms/wings.
- **Sandbag:**
  - Lie down and imagine you're a sandbag. Now roll over, using the least amount of effort possible.
- **Psoas release:**
  - On your back, with knees bent, slowly slide the right heel forward to straighten the leg and squeeze the buttock muscles. Slowly return to the left foot and switch sides.
- **Earth Breathing:**
  - Let yourself melt into the earth with each exhalation and gradually imagine that your bodily rhythms are merging with the energy of the earth.

Daily Lesson Plan #49
Anxiety Calming Movement Practice

Intention/Objective
This is a sample class from Anxiety Recovery Training
Teaching Resource Material
Soft music, eye pillow, and a band for each student.
Review/Introduction
Everyone feels anxious occasionally, because anxiety is a normal experience. Our kids may worry when faced with an important event, a challenging exam, or preparing for a performance. But anxiety disorders are different. They're considered a group of mental illnesses that cause constant and overwhelming fear, stress and disruption. Excessive anxiety can cause students to avoid school, their jobs, family gatherings, and other social situations that might trigger or worsen their symptoms. While they start as coping strategies for surviving stressful times, anxiety behaviours lead to harmful symptoms in the long term.
Lesson
The following is a practice to help break the anxiety cycle and find calm in body and mind. Move slowly and be guided by your growing edge. • Childs or Puppy, letting head rest on a block or on hands. • Table with barrel rolls, rolling the ribcage in one direction, then the other • Quad Stretch, on abdomen, one leg at a time • Superhero, like the locust but with arms lifted and outstretched • Downward Facing Dog, letting the head dangle freely • Forward Fold, inviting the neck to lengthen • Palm activation - rub palms together by spinning hands in opposite directions. Once heat is created, rest your hands over the eyes to release tension headaches. Rub the hands together again, this time resting hands on a body part that needs extra support. • Cloud hands - see Trauma-sensitive practice above • Fearless Heart (Hridaya) Mudra, at the heart, with backs of the hands together, interlock pinkies, ring fingers and index fingers. Join middle finger and thumbs together and breathe to release fear, anxiety and stress from the heart. • Savasana/Relaxation with lower legs on a chair. Apply your eye pillow and practice 1:2 ratio breathing.

Daily Lesson Plan #50: Wrap up

Intention/Objective
Review of main teachings in a playful game of Jeopardy and a worksheet.
Teaching Resource Material
<ul><li>Game of Jeopardy Outline</li><li>Yoga 11 Worksheet</li></ul>
Review/Introduction
Student led session using posters - 10 minutes.
Lesson
Review course content through the Game of Jeopardy and the Yoga 11 Worksheet.
Reflection/Conclusion
<ul><li>Discuss Stephen Covey's 8th habit for highly successful people - discovering and expressing your inner voice. The teachings of Yoga are now in their hands, not just to live them but to share them with the world.</li><li>Finish with optional Hugasana, or group hug and share appreciation for anyone who's helped you through this yoga journey.</li></ul>

Game of Jeopardy

Three points if answered correctly, one point if given to the other team and answered correctly, minus one if the wrong answer is given.

1. What is the meaning of Yoga? Union of mind, body, spirit.
2. How old is Yoga? 5,000 yrs old.
3. Yoga's sounding breath in the back of the throat is called? Ujjayi Pranayama/Breathing.
4. The system of engaging muscular locks is called? Bandhas.
5. What does the term drishti mean? Eye gaze.
6. Demonstrate an asana that strengthens the triceps? Shoulder Pressing/Bhujapidasana or Crow/Bakasana.
7. The anatomical name for the kneecap is…Patella.
8. Where do the quadriceps live on the body? the upper leg.
9. List two systems of the body. Circulatory, digestive, nervous, muscular, skeletal, immune system etc.
10. Should Yoga be done on a full stomach? Why or why not…no.
11. Name one of the Yamas and its meaning…
12. Name one of the Niyamas and its meaning…
13. Demonstrate an asana whose foundation is with the feet parallel to one another, (for example: Prasarita Padottanasana or Padangusthasana), have them demonstrate.
14. What balance asana opens the hips? Ardha Chandrasana (demonstrate).
15. What is the English translation for this asana: Utthita Parsvakonasana and demonstrate? Extended Side Angle.
16. Who is known as the author of the Yoga Sutra? Patanjali.
17. What are the Sanskrit words for hands and feet? Hastas and padas (double points).
18. What is the Sanskrit word for loving kindness practice? Metta.
19. What is the translation of Namaste? The light in me bows to the light in you.
20. What does Shanti mean? Peace.

Daily Lesson Plan #50: Wrap up

Yoga 11 Worksheet

1. The most effective way to learn yoga is:
   a. Through a video
   b. At an all-inclusive resort with friends
   c. By studying philosophy
   d. Through regular practice with the guidance of an experienced teacher
2. The most common type of yoga practiced in the west is...

3. What does this popular type of yoga translate to in English?

Origins and Philosophy

1. Where did the practice of Yoga originate?

2. How old is Yoga?

3. The language of Yoga is_____.

4. Name the two main texts in yoga and the translation of their titles:
   a.
   b.

Physical Practice

1. The term Ayurveda means_____.

2. What's your dosha? List three personal characteristics that describe this dosha, and you.

3. An ideal yoga class unfolds in phases. The three main aspects of a general class are:

4. What does Surya Namaskar mean?

5. What does Vinyasa mean?

6. The yogic translation for Extended Triangle is_____.

7. What type of breathing is best during asana practice? _____

Mindfulness

1. List four benefits of living mindfully.
   a.
   b.
   c.
   d.

2. When stress hijacks a person's body, what division of the Autonomic Nervous System becomes aroused?

3. What are three signs of the stress response?

Personal Reflection

1. What is the greatest lesson you've gained from your yoga practice so far?

2. At this point on your journey, what aspect of yoga do you need to focus most on?

Breathing Practices included in this Manual

Teaching Considerations

- **Environment:** Ensure a calm, quiet space for most breath practices.
- **Contraindications:** Always screen for contraindications prior to teaching advanced breathwork.
- **Progression:** Introduce breath practices gradually; allow students to develop comfort and skill before progressing.
- **Integration:** Breath practices may be used as stand-alone techniques or woven into asana, meditation, and mindfulness classes.

Yogic Breathing is a smooth, natural, and health-enhancing way of breathing that engages all three chambers of the lungs. On the inhale, the breath expands the belly, rises through the chest, and lifts the collarbones. On the exhale, the collarbones, chest, and belly gently deflate in reverse order. This full, mindful breath nourishes the body and calms the nervous system.

Balloon Breathing is another name for Yogic Breathing, using the image of a balloon to guide the breath, making it suitable for diverse learners or young students. As the lungs expand and deflate like a balloon, students are invited to imagine the color and size of their balloon, which can shift with each practice. This playful visualization not only enhances breath awareness but also helps students tune into the state of their chest—revealing how open, free, or tense it feels based on how easily their "balloon" inflates.

Empowered Breathing is the style of breath used during physical activity. It emphasizes diaphragmatic expansion and contraction primarily in the ribcage area. It is not as deep as the full Yogic Breath because of the engagement of the *bandhas* in the pelvic floor and lower abdomen, which provide core stability and internal support during movement.

Ujjayi Breathing, also referred to as "Victorious Breath", "Ocean Breathing," or even "Darth Vadar Breathing" is a foundational pranayama technique used to create focus, warmth, and steadiness in the body and mind. It involves gently constricting the back of the throat (glottis) to create a soft, whisper-like sound as you inhale and exhale through the nose. This audible breath helps to harness attention, regulate the nervous system, and build internal heat—making it especially useful during asana practice.

Bee Breathing (*Bhramari Pranayama*) involves inhaling gently through the nose and exhaling with a soft, humming sound—like the gentle buzz of a bee. This vibrational sound activates the vagus nerve, helping to calm the nervous system, reduce stress, and quiet the mind. Practicing Bee Breathing regularly can soothe the arousal system and promote a deep sense of inner peace.

Fall-Out Breaths are a simple and effective way to release tension from the body. This technique involves inhaling through the nose and exhaling through the mouth with a sigh—either voiced or breathy. It's especially helpful for students experiencing stress, frustration, or agitation, as it allows for an immediate release of pent-up energy. This breath is not meant to be sustained over long periods; typically, three rounds are enough to create a noticeable shift. Fall-Out Breathing pairs well with dynamic practices like **Breath of Joy**, offering a grounding way to settle after stimulation.

1:2 Ratio Breathing refers to the relationship between the length of the inhale and the exhale. The "1" represents the in-breath (e.g., a 4-count inhale), and the "2" represents an exhale that is twice as long (e.g., an 8-count exhale). This simple yet powerful breathing technique is deeply calming. By extending the exhale, it activates the parasympathetic nervous system, helping to quiet the fight-or-flight response and guide the body into a state of rest and relaxation.

Alternate Nostril Breathing (*Nadi Shodhana*) is a more advanced form of breathwork that involves breathing in and out through one nostril at a time, using the fingers to gently close off each side. Typically, the breath is held briefly at the top of each inhale to deepen the calming effects. By balancing the left and right hemispheres of the brain, this practice helps to regulate the nervous system and promote inner harmony.

Kapalabhati Breathing, also known as *"Skull-Shining Breath"* or *bellows breathing*, is an advanced breathwork technique that involves a series of passive inhalations, followed by sharp, forceful exhalations through the nose. The focus is on the exhalation, with the abdominal muscles actively pumping to expel the breath. This energizing practice helps to clear stagnant or unhealthy energy, stimulate digestion, and restore the body's natural breathing rhythm. It should not be practiced, however, by pregnant students or those with high blood pressure.

Breathing Practices Overview

Note: Unless otherwise indicated, these breathing techniques are generally practiced in Maitryasana (Friendship Pose) or Sukhasana (Easy Pose).

Breath Practice	Technique Description	Teaching Notes & Benefits
Yogic Breathing	Full breath engaging the lower belly, chest, and collarbones. Inhale: belly expands → chest rises → collarbones lift. Exhale: reverse order.	Foundational breath for calming the nervous system, nourishing the body, and cultivating mindfulness.
Balloon Breathing	Uses the image of a balloon to guide breath expansion and release. Students visualize their balloon inflating and deflating.	Supports breath awareness through visualization; ideal for children and diverse learners; integrates emotional awareness.
Empowered Breathing	Ribcage-focused diaphragmatic breath with subtle engagement of the pelvic floor and lower abdominal bandhas.	Supports physical activity, movement, and stability. Bandha engagement provides core support while maintaining breath flow.
Ujjayi Breathing ("Victorious Breath")	Gentle glottis constriction creates a soft whisper-like sound as breath flows through the nose.	Builds focus, steadiness, and internal warmth; regulates nervous system; enhances presence during asana practice.
Bee Breathing (Bhramari Pranayama)	Inhale gently; exhale with a soft humming or buzzing sound through the nose.	Activates the vagus nerve; soothes the nervous system; quiets the mind; reduces anxiety and mental agitation.
Fall-Out Breaths	Inhale through the nose, exhale through the mouth with a voiced or breathy sigh. Typically repeated for 3 rounds.	Quick tension release; helps transition from agitation or stimulation to calm; pairs well with dynamic sequences.
1:2 Ratio Breathing	Exhale duration is twice as long as inhale (e.g., 4-count inhale, 8-count exhale).	Deeply calming; activates the parasympathetic nervous system; supports downregulation and rest.

Daily Lesson Plan #50: Wrap up

Alternate Nostril Breathing (Nadi Shodhana)	Breath alternates between nostrils, closing one nostril at a time; brief breath retention may be included.	Balances left/right brain hemispheres; regulates energy; promotes internal harmony and nervous system balance.
Kapalabhati Breathing ("Skull Shining Breath")	Passive inhale; sharp, forceful exhale through nose with active abdominal contractions.	Energizes body; clears stagnation; stimulates digestion. Contraindications: Avoid during pregnancy and with hypertension.

"In yoga, we learn to create space where we once felt stuck. To unfold layers of protection we've built around our hearts."— Unknown

50 Foundational Asanas

These asanas have been thoughtfully selected based on key principles to support a safe, accessible, and empowering yoga practice:

- **To establish a strong foundation** for progression into more advanced postures over time.
- **To prioritize joint safety**, avoiding high-risk postures such as Wheel (*Urdhva Dhanurasana*), and emphasizing alignment.
- **To ensure accessibility** for a wide range of students, including variations using a chair to support diverse needs.
- **To open the front body and strengthen the back**, using gentle backbends and core engagement to improve posture and spinal health.
- **To counteract the effects of prolonged sitting**, by incorporating hip openers and strength-building postures that support functional movement.
- **To create a trauma-sensitive environment**, focusing on postures that promote autonomy and emotional safety (while omitting potentially triggering shapes like Ananda Balasanda).
- **To encourage playfulness and joy**, with expressive asanas such as *Wild Thing* that invite creative movement and self-expression.

"Each time you show up on your mat, you are growing stronger — not just in body, but in mind and heart." — Unknown

Daily Lesson Plan #50: Wrap up

Mindfulness Asanas

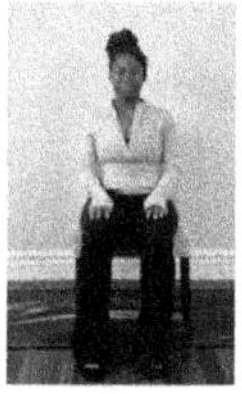 Friendship Asana/ *Maitryasana*	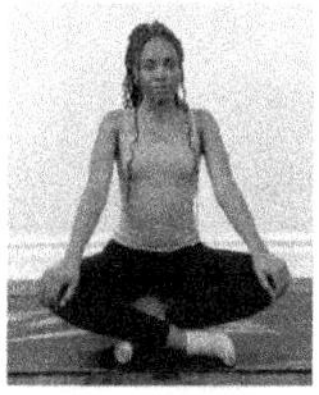 Easy Asana/ *Sukhasana*	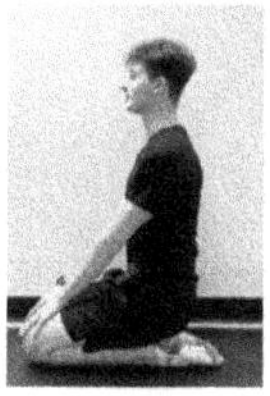 Hero/ *Virasana*	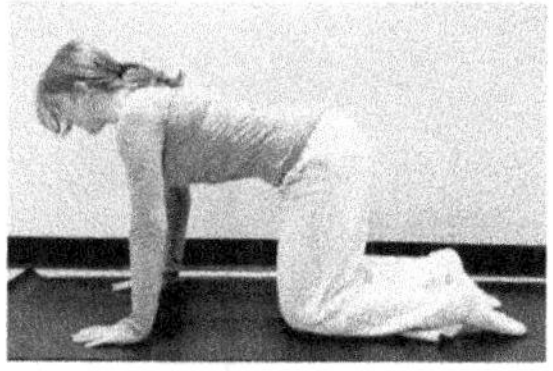 Table A/ *Bharmanasana A*
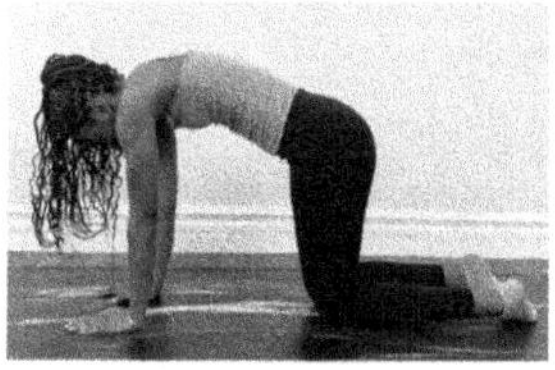 Table B/ *Bharmanasana B*	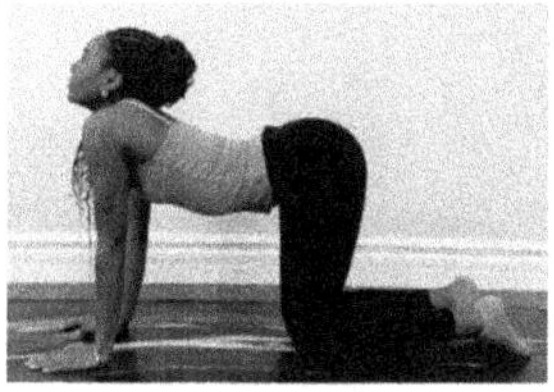 Table C/ *Bharmanasana C*	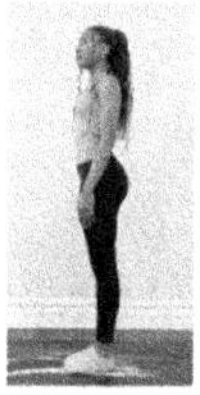 Mountain/ *Tadasana*	

Standing Asanas

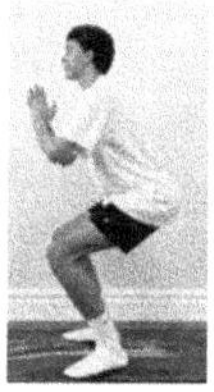 Powerful Asana A/ *Utkatasana A*	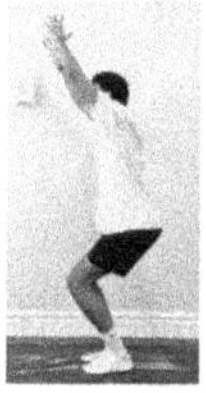 Powerful Asana B/ *Utkatasana B*	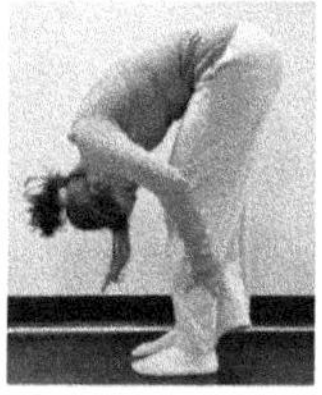 Standing Forward Fold/ *Padangusthasana*	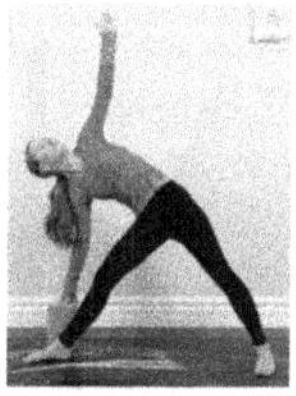 Extended Triangle/ *Utthita Trikonasana*
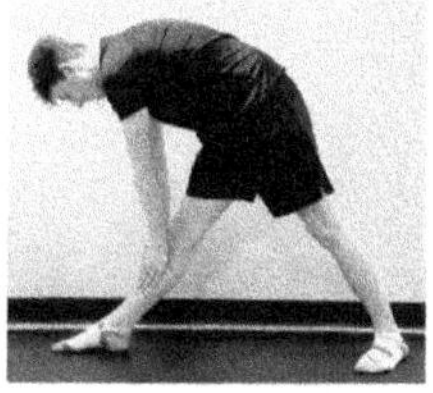 Side Intense Stretch/ *Parsvottanasana*	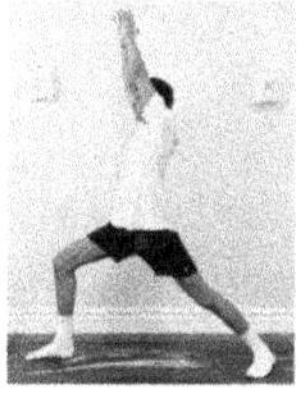 Warrior 1/ *Virabhadrasana 1*	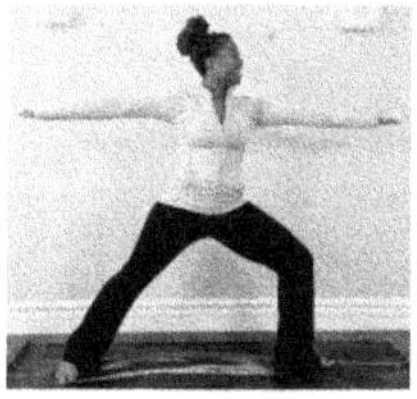 Warrior 2/ *Virabhadrasana 2*	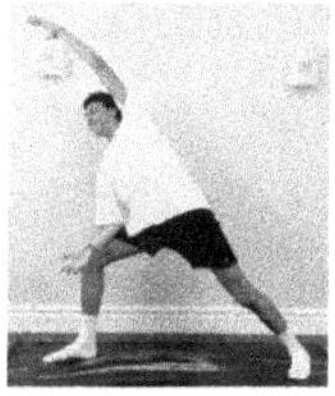 Extended Side Angle A/ *Utthita Parsvakonasana A*
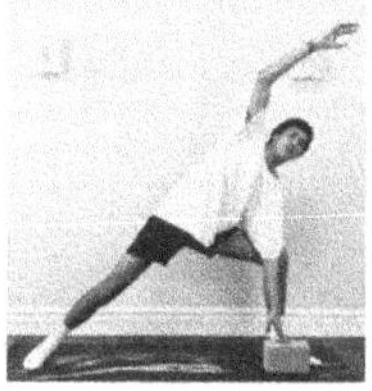 Extended Side Angle B/ *Utthita Parsvakonasana B*	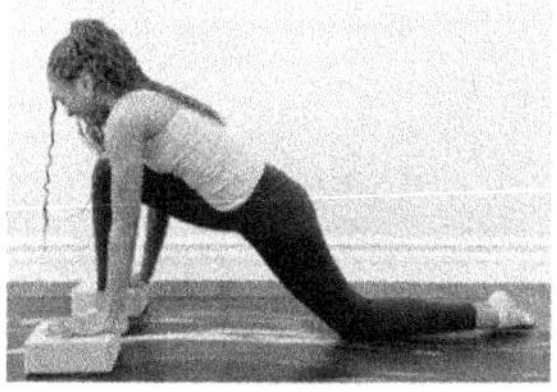 Lunge A/ *Anjaneyasana A*	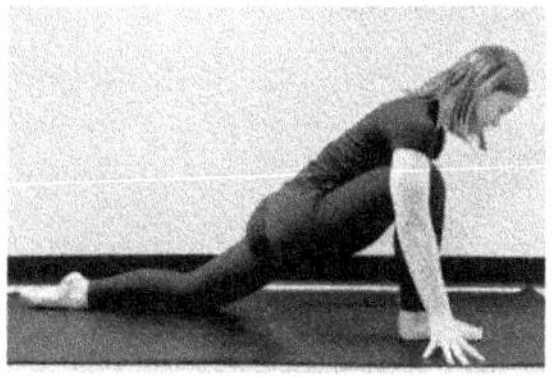 Lunge B/ *Anjaneyasana B*	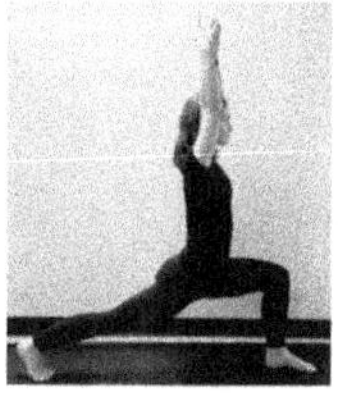 Lunge C/ *Anjaneyasana C*

Standing Balance Asanas

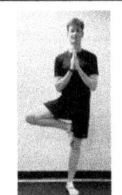 Tree A/ *Vrksasana A*	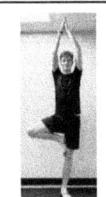 Tree B/ *Vrksasana B*	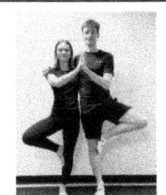 Partner Tree/ *Partner Vrksasana*	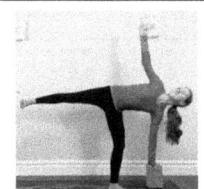 Standing Half Moon Balance/ *Ardha Chandrasana*
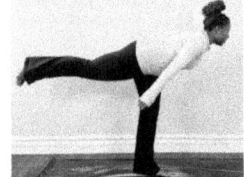 Warrior 3A/ *Virabhadrasana 3A*	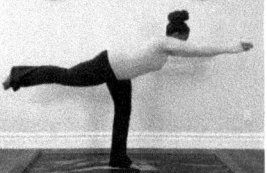 Warrior 3B/ *Virabhadrasana 3B*	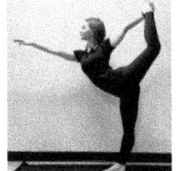 Dancer/ *Natarajasana*	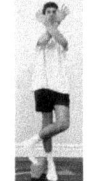 Eagle A/ *Garudasana A*
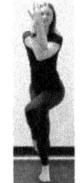 Eagle B/ *Garudasana B*			

Arm Balance Asanas

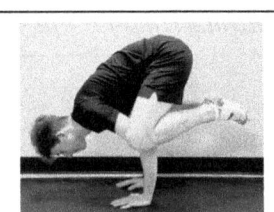 The Crow/ *Bakasana*	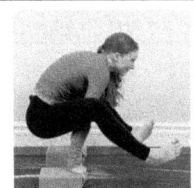 Shoulder Pressing Asana A/ *Bhujapidasana A*	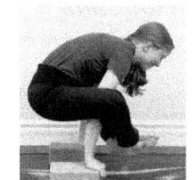 Shoulder Pressing Asana B/ *Bhujapidasana B*

Inversions

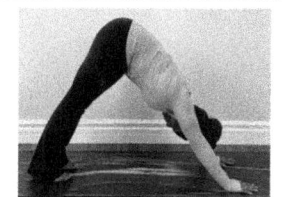	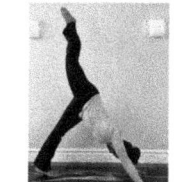	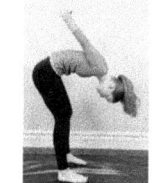	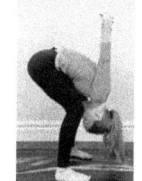
Downward Facing Dog A/*Adho Mukha Svanasana A*	Downward Facing Dog B/*Adho Mukha Svanasana B*	Yoga Mudra A/ *Interlocking Fingers A*	Yoga Mudra B/ *Interlocking Fingers B*

Backbending Asanas

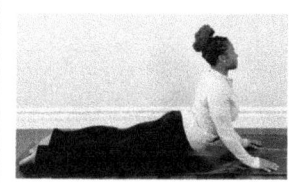	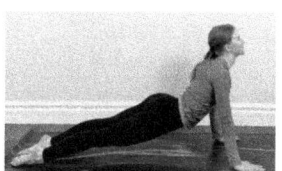	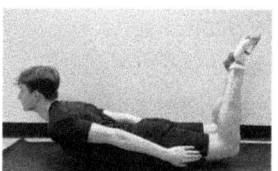	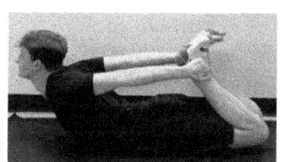
Cobra/ *Bhujangasana*	Upward Facing Dog/ *Urdhva Mukha Svanasana*	Bow A/ *Dhanurasana A*	Bow B/ *Dhanurasana B*
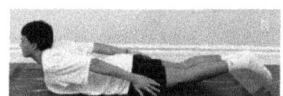	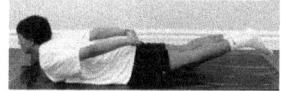	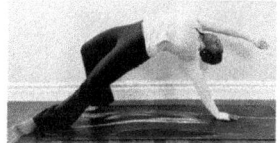	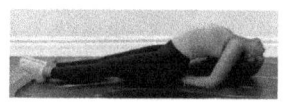
Locust A/ *Shalabhasana A*	Locust B/ *Shalabhasana B*	Wild Thing/ *Camatkarasana*	Fish/ *Matsyasana*

Seated Asanas

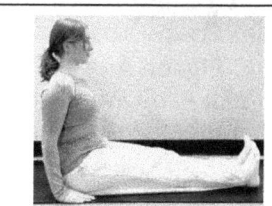	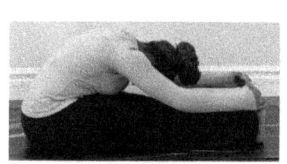	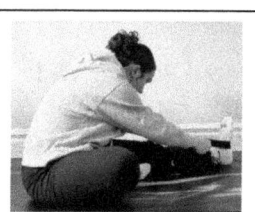
Seated Staff/ *Dandasana*	Seated Forward Fold/ *Paschimottanasana*	Head to Knee/ *Janu Sirsasana*

Core Strengthening Asanas

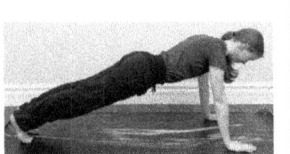 High Plank/ Plankasana/ *Kumbhakasana*	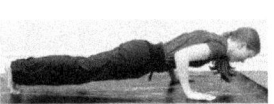 Four Limbed Staff/ *Chaturanga Dandasana*	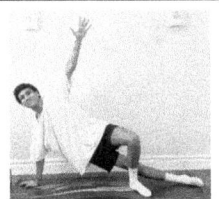 Side Plank A/ *Vasisthasana A*	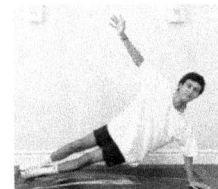 Side Plank B/ *Vasisthasana B*
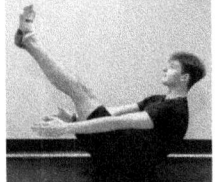 Full Boat/ *Paripurna Navasana*	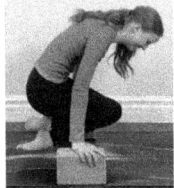 Scale Asana A/ *Lolasana A*	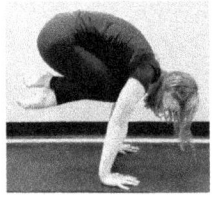 Scale Asana B/ *Lolasana B*	

Hip Opening Asanas

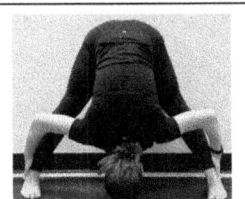 Standing Wide Angle Forward Fold/ *Prasarita Padottanasana*	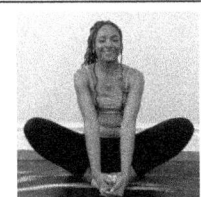 Bound Angle A/ *Baddha Konasana A*	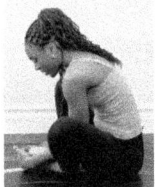 Bound Angle B/ *Baddha Konasana B*	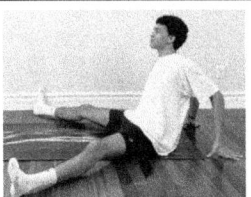 Seated Wide Angle Forward Fold A/ *Upavistha Konasana A*
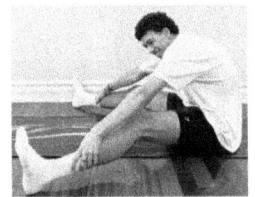 Seated Wide Angle Forward Fold B/ *Upavistha Konasana B*	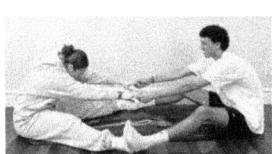 Seated Partner Wide Angle Forward Fold/ *Upavistha Konasana*	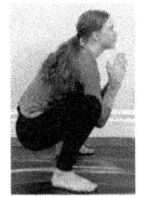 Yogic Squat/ *Malasana*	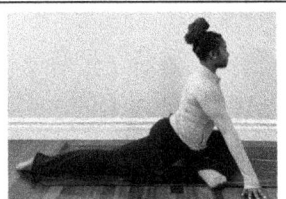 Pigeon A/ *Eka Pada Raja Kapotasana A*
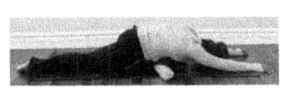 Pigeon B/ *Eka Pada Raja Kapotasana B*	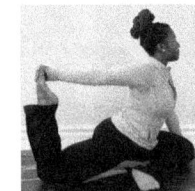 Pigeon C/ *Eka Pada Raja Kapotasana C*	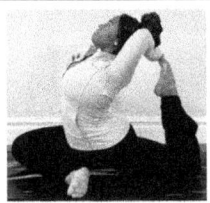 Pigeon D/ *Eka Pada Raja Kapotasana D*	

Daily Lesson Plan #50: Wrap up

Twisting Asanas

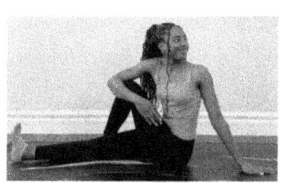 Seated Twist A/*Ardha Matsyendrasana A*	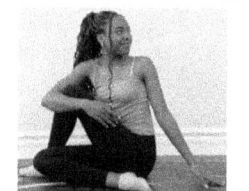 Seated Twist B/*Ardha Matsyendrasana B*	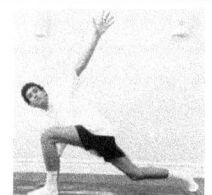 Revolved Side Angle/*Parivrtta Parsvakonasana*	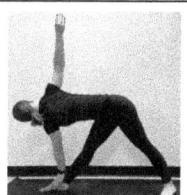 Revolved Triangle/*Parivrtta Trikonasana*
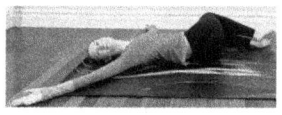 Supine Twist/*Jathara Parivartanasana*			

Closing Asanas

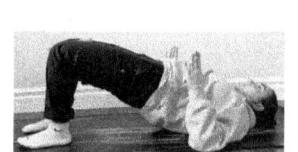 Half Bridge A/ *Setu Bandhasana A*	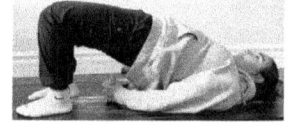 Half Bridge B/ *Setu Bandhasana B*	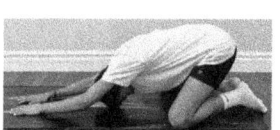 Child's/ *Balasana*	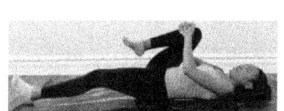 Knee to Chest A/ *Apanasana A*
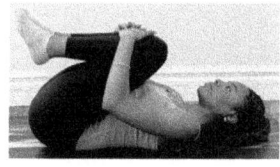 Knees to Chest B/ *Apanasana B*	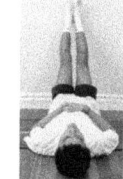 Legs Up the Wall A/ *Viparita Karani A*	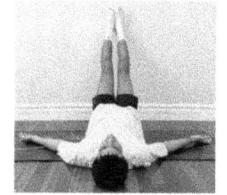 Legs Up the Wall B/ *Viparita Karani B*	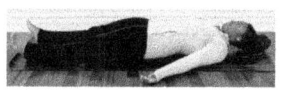 Corpse/Relaxation/ *Savasana*

"Yoga is not about touching your toes. It is what you learn on the way down." — Jigar Gor

www.ingramcontent.com/pod-product-compliance
Lightning Source LLC
Chambersburg PA
CBHW081157020426
42333CB00020B/2531